Bike Healthy

How cycling will help you look good, feel good and quite possibly live longer.

by Peter Andrews

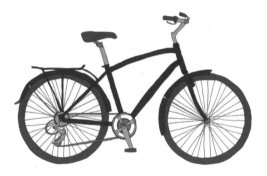

Illustrations by Hannah Broadway

ISBN: 978-0-9927248-1-8

Safety first!

The author, publisher and distributor of Bike Healthy advise readers to take full responsibility for their safety and to know their limits. Before practising any of the exercises or activities in this book be sure that your cycle and related equipment are fully fit for purpose. Do not take risks beyond your level of ability, experience, aptitude, training and fitness. The exercises and activities in this book are not intended as substitutes for those prescribed by your doctor or other health professional. As with all exercise, you should get your doctor's approval before beginning.

Disclaimer:

Whilst every effort has been made to ensure the accuracy of the information in this book the author and publisher accept no responsibility for any errors or omissions. Occasionally, the book mentions particular brands, products or services by name. This is for information only. The author does not recommend or endorse particular companies and nobody has paid anything to get a mention in Bike Healthy!

Note:

Bike Healthy follows on from an earlier book, first published in 2008, called Bike Easy: Top Tips and Expert Advice for the New Cyclist and it shares some of the content. The chapters on buying a bike, getting it set up for ease of use and comfort, and choosing suitable clothing and cycling accessories are similar. You really only need one book or the other, not both. However, if you want a copy of Bike Easy it's still available from all good book stores or direct from the publisher www.ParkThatBike.com

Published by
ParkThatBike
14 The Barracks
Parkend
Gloucestershire GL15 4HR
www.ParkThatBike.com

Printed and bound in the UK by Russell Press
www.russellpress.com
Printed on recycled paper

Peter Andrews is a lifelong environmentalist, a seven-day-a-week cyclist, an entrepreneur and a professional cycling advocate. For 20 years, in both the charitable and the private sectors, he has worked on initiatives to encourage everyday cycling including Bikeability training programmes, cycle maintenance courses, bike parking schemes, and cycling for health projects. Peter's previous book Bike Easy: Top Tips & Expert Advice for the New Cyclist has been used by local councils across the UK to support their cycling development programmes. Peter lives in the heart of the Forest of Dean with an assortment of bikes and a tandem.

www.parkthatbike.com

Dr Adrian Davis is internationally recognised as an expert in the field of transport and health. He has worked in academia, for a commercial transport consultancy, and for UK local authorities. He authored the British Medical Association's first Transport Policy report in 1997, and has written reports for the World Health Organisation and UK cycling organisations. In 2012-13 Adrian worked in the Department for Transport's Sustainable Transport Directorate to provide public health support. He drafted a report on the economic value of active travel interventions which was published in 2014. He is an Assistant Editor of the Journal of Transport and Health, and a Visiting Professor at the University of the West of England.

www.dradriandavis.wordpress.com

Hannah Broadway has worked as an illustrator for over a decade, with a range of clients from the NHS to Bristol University to Bloomsbury Publishing. She has illustrated five picture books, designed T-shirts for Mild West Heroes, done a big old mural for Bristol's Harbourside, "popped up" with Made in Bristol as a guest artist, and knows just how lucky she is to do a job she loves! Hannah lives in Bristol with her husband, little girl and two cats. She is learning to grow vegetables, trying to get better at cycling up hills and continues to enjoy making it up as she goes along!

www.hannah-broadway-pictures.blogspot.com

Contents

Foreword : "It's not rocket science…"

For 30 years, working with bodies such as the World Health Organisation, the Departments of Health and Transport in England, Public Health England, numerous UK local authorities, and voluntary sector organisations including Sustrans and the CTC, I have been researching physically active forms of travel. The research evidence from across the world is absolutely clear: even though there is no such thing as a "wonder drug", physical activity comes remarkably close because of its multiple benefits. Its anti-inflammatory properties protect us against the development of serious conditions such as heart disease and stroke and even some cancers. Consequently, it lowers the risk of illness and of premature death. And, in addition, it reduces stress and makes us feel good.

It is not rocket science that one of the best ways to incorporate physical activity into your life is through cycling. Not only will it lower your stress levels and keep you well; it also gets you to your destination leaving more money in your pocket for the nicer things in life while not adding to climate change. More cycling means healthier individuals, vibrant communities, and a fitter, more resilient nation.

Objective measurement, rather than self-reporting, reveals that 95% of adults in England do not achieve the minimum of 150 minutes a week of physical activity recommended by Chief Medical Officers. In fact, in our busy and technology-driven lives, we have fairly successfully eliminated most forms of physical activity, or at least risk doing so. This is a major concern for public health specialists like me who want to improve the fitness and well-being of the population. It also has serious implications for NHS expenditure, businesses efficiency, and the strength of the economy.

Cycling should be a normal everyday transport choice for most of the population, from the youngest to the eldest. Yet levels of cycle use in Britain are low. As a nation we currently make only 3% of our journeys by bike, despite the fact that 61 percent of trips are less than five miles in length.[1]

Happily, things are changing and there are encouraging signs. There are many

---

1   Department for Transport. 2013. National Travel Survey: 2012. [Online]. [Accessed 18 December 2014]. Available from: https://www.gov.uk/government/uploads/system/uploads/attachment_data/file/243957/nts2012-01.pdf

examples of good practice and enlightened leadership, both from continental Europe and increasingly from within the UK. My home city of Bristol, for example, has invested in cycling and has doubled the number of people who commute by bike between 2001 and 2011, according to census surveys. Cycling now accounts for 10 percent of journeys to work.[2] And cycle use continues to grow in many UK towns and cities as more people recognise the multiple benefits of choosing the bike.

Cycling really can change lives. If people are to make the change they need support, encouragement and practical help. This book provides exactly that! I'm delighted to endorse it.

Dr Adrian Davis FFPH
Visiting Professor, University of the West of England
Associate Editor, Journal of Transport & Health

---

2   2011 Office of National Statistics census figures.

Introduction : Welcome!

In environmental circles there's a wise old saying that runs as a mini-question and answer session. It goes like this:
Q. When is the best time to plant a tree?
A. Thirty years ago.
Q. When is the second best time to plant a tree?
A. Now.

It's exactly the same with health. In a perfect world we'd all eat a perfect diet and get regular exercise from the day we take our first baby steps. We'd breathe nothing but fresh mountain air and drink only spring water.

Alas, real life isn't like that and many people find themselves out of condition, overweight or unwell because of their lifestyle choices, their genetic inheritance, or through sheer bad luck. We can't turn the clock back, but, as with the tree planting analogy, the key is to act now. If you do, it can have a massive effect on your health and well-being.

If you've made decision to be more active, then your best friend is your bike! All forms of physical activity have their merits, but cycling is uniquely beneficial. Just about anybody can do it, you can integrate it into your life, the financial costs are low, and the health benefits are far-reaching. Your muscles and joints, your cardiovascular system, even your mind and spirit will feel the difference. It can defend your body against problems such as heart disease, stroke and cancer, or, for people already afflicted, it can help stabilise or, often, improve the condition.

I realise that, for lots of people, it takes real courage to get onto a bike, or to get back onto it if you've lost the cycling habit. Today's roads can look daunting and modern bikes, to say nothing of all the accessories and the lurid apparel, can be off-putting to many. Rest assured, it really isn't that hard! You don't have to wear Lycra if you don't want to. You don't have to ride at a breakneck speed on a bike that cost three months wages. You don't even have to cycle every day to yield the health benefits. And cycling should never hurt! On the contrary it should be a pleasant – delightful, even – experience. Bike Healthy explains how.

It explains why cycling is such a good form of exercise. It covers buying a bike, kitting it out, and achieving comfort while riding it. It helps you find the best places to ride, and it prepares you for real-life journeys, whether for leisure and pleasure or for practical purposes such as shopping and commuting. And, because life doesn't always go as planned, there's a whole chapter of tips that will help you stay keen and motivated.

Think of Bike Healthy as your personal guidebook. You might be a fit person who simply wants to get more out of their cycling and stay in a good shape. You might be out of shape and planning to improve your health. You might be someone with a medical condition who's been advised to take more exercise. Whatever your needs and aspirations you'll find something helpful in Bike Healthy.

Peter Andrews

The perfect exercise

Human beings are built for movement. Our lean, fit, hunter-gatherer ancestors were always on the go, roaming across vast distances, intrigued by and interacting with their environment. Later, when we settled down and invented agriculture, we roped in animals to help us and we invented simple machines such as water wheels; but most of the hard work was still done by hand. Much of the landscape we see around us today was shaped by human muscle.

The industrial revolution saw us harness steam power and develop complex machinery but, for most people, work was still something physical. Around the home there was coal to heave, wood to chop, carpets to be beaten, floors to sweep and laundry to be pummelled in a dolly tub. In the garden there was earth to be turned and lawns to be raked, rolled and mown. All of these tasks were done manually.

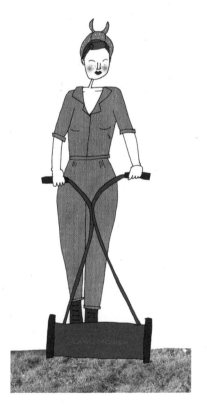

Fast forward to the early twenty-first century and it's a very different picture. Our workplaces are crammed with sophisticated technology and many processes are automated. Our hi-tech homes are filled with labour-saving devices and we use cars or public transport for even the shortest trips. When it comes to recreation, that's increasingly home-based too; we settle down in front of our TVs or computers and live life through the feelings and actions of other people. We're content to let someone else do the ballroom dancing, kick a ball, or give their garden a makeover.

Now, to many people, myself included, this doesn't sound too unpleasant. Who doesn't enjoy reclining on the sofa with a glass of something and a good programme on the telly? The trouble is, although it's fine in moderation, the sedentary lifestyle has become the norm. It's making us fat, and it's making us unwell. The number of people in the UK who are overweight or obese has more than trebled in the last 25 years (it's now 61% of adults and 30% of children)[3] and serious health problems such as heart disease, stroke, diabetes and cancer have increased sharply.

According to the Department of Health, adults need at least 150 minutes of "moderate intensity physical activity" every week to maintain good health. Ideally, the moderate exercise will be supplemented by periodic bouts of more vigorous activity, enough to speed up your breathing without leaving you gasping. You should also include some activities that strengthen the body's major muscles.[4]

How much physical activity do we need?

To stay healthy, adults (that's people aged 19 to 64) should try to be active daily for at least 10 minutes every day and should complete 150 minutes (2 hours and 30 minutes) of moderate-intensity aerobic activity every week. For example: an easy paced bike ride.

OR
75 minutes (1 hour and 15 minutes) of vigorous-intensity aerobic activity every week. For example: a briskly paced bike ride.

PLUS
Whether you go for the moderate or the vigorous option, you should also do some muscle-strengthening activities on at least 2 days a week. These are actions that exercise the major muscle groups (legs, hips, back, abdomen, chest, shoulders and arms) repeatedly, to the point where it becomes a struggle. Cycling up a lengthy hill works the leg muscles nicely.

REMEMBER
• These levels of activity are ideals. If you're unfit or if you've been unwell it might take a while before you can achieve them.
• It's fine to do a mixture of the two options to suit your mood and the time available.
• Older people (aged 65 and over) should also aim to achieve these levels of physical activity – and it's never too late to start. Take extra care if you have weak legs, poor balance or a medical condition. You might also benefit from some preparatory exercises to improve your balance and co-ordination.
• Children and young people need considerably more physical activity. (See Chapter Two.)
• Freewheeling, waiting at traffic lights or sitting in tea shops doesn't count towards your activity total. You have to be pedalling!

---

3   Department of Health and Ellison, J. MP. 2013. *Reducing obesity and improving diet.* [Online]. [Accessed 5 January 2015]. Available from: https://www.gov.uk/government/policies/reducing-obesity-and-improving-diet

4   NHS choices. 2013. *Physical activity guidelines for adults.* [Online]. [Accessed 6 January 2015]. Available from: http://www.nhs.uk/Livewell/fitness/Pages/physical-activity-guidelines-for-adults.aspx

Jogging, canoeing, swimming, dance classes, sessions on gym apparatus such as treadmills and rowing machines are all fine forms of physical activity, so too are everyday activities such as gardening and DIY so long as they're done frequently and with a certain amount of vigour. But if you had to choose just one form of physical activity, it's hard to beat cycling. Here are some of its advantages:

- **Cycling is accessible to almost everyone.** Apart from a bike and a few accessories you need no specialised equipment.
- **Cycling can be incorporated into your daily routine and done pretty much all the year round.** If you cycle to work, for example, there's your exercise for the day.
- **Cycling can be done at various intensities.** It meets health experts' requirements for both moderate- and vigorous-intensity aerobic forms of exercise, and every time you heave yourself up a hill that's a muscle strengthening form of exercise too. A typical bike ride incorporates lots of natural resting moments, when you freewheel downhill for example, and this combination of action followed by rest enables you to keep going for a considerable period of time without feeling tired.
- **Cycling is gentle on your joints.** Unlike anything that involves running or jumping there's no shock to the joints. This is particularly helpful if you are overweight or if you have problems such as arthritis.
- **Cycling is sociable.** You can ride on your own or do it with family members or friends. Joining a club or going on an organised ride can be a great way to meet new people and widen your social circle.
- **And cycling is fun!** It's about independence and freedom, breathing fresh air, savouring the sights, sounds and smells of the countryside. It's about being in control of the journey, setting the pace and deciding the route, delighting in an unexpected detour, a chance encounter or a new discovery.

One of the major benefits of cycling is that it can help you lose weight. Being close to your proper body weight has been proved to be a crucial factor in warding off ill health. According to the National Institute for Health and Care Excellence (NICE), most people who need to lose weight can get health benefits from losing even a small amount – about 5% – of their excess weight.[5] Riding a bicycle at a moderate pace uses up 300 to 400 calories an hour.

---

5   NHS choices. 2013. *What are the benefits of losing weight?* [Online]. [Accessed 5 January 2015]. Available from: http://www.nhs.uk/chq/Pages/848.aspx?CategoryID=51&SubCategoryID=165

How do you size up?

Doctors use the body mass index (BMI) as a simple way of assessing whether a patient needs to lose weight. The calculation is based on comparing a person's weight with their body height. It applies equally to men and women. Find out whether you're a healthy weight for your height by using the table below.

Another easy way to get an insight into your health and weight is to measure your waistline. It should be no longer than half your height. A study based on two decades of medical research, suggests that a waist to height ratio of 80 percent or more could reduce your life expectancy by up to 20 years.[6] Waist circumference is important because it shows the amount of central or visceral fat in the body which is linked to high cholesterol, diabetes and heart disease.

Six feet (72 inches) tall? Your waistline should be 36 inches or, preferably, less. Five feet (60 inches) tall? 30 inches or less. You get the idea. Now, fetch the tape measure!

Combined with sensible eating, regular cycling is likely to mean that you lose some weight and keep it off. Cycling has the added benefit of ramping up your metabolism so that, even after the ride is over, you continue to burn up fat. Losing that excess weight will make you look and feel better and can reduce your risk of developing some serious health problems including:

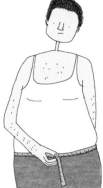

- high blood pressure
- heart disease
- stroke
- type 2 diabetes
- colon and breast cancer
- osteoarthritis
- back pain
- depression and anxiety

If you've already got one of these conditions cycling can still be of benefit as a way of controlling it and, possibly, reducing it. We look at cycling as a form of therapy in Chapter Nine.

6   The Telegraph. 2014. *Key to a long life is a waist measuring less than half your height.* [Online]. [Accessed 5 January 2015]. Available from: http://www.telegraph.co.uk/health/11080588/Key-to-a-long-life-is-a-waist-measuring-less-than-half-your-height.html

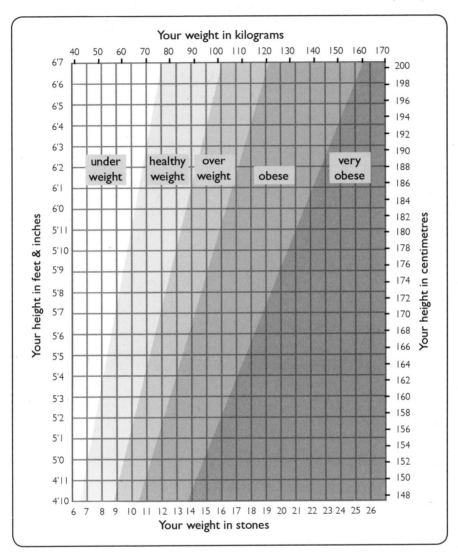

Your weight in kilograms

Your height in feet & inches / Your height in centimetres

under weight | healthy weight | over weight | obese | very obese

Your weight in stones

As well as warding off future problems, cycling will improve your health in the here and now. Here are the top five benefits:

Muscles : Cycling strengthens your body's largest muscles. Your quadriceps and hamstrings in the upper leg, and the gastrocnemius and soleus in the calf all work in a sequence to perform the pedalling action that moves you forward. Exercising these muscles leads to an increase in stamina and strength, and better posture. Done

13

properly (see Chapter Eight), pedalling is a light, repetitive action with little risk of over-exercise or strain.

You might not expect cycling to do much for your top half, but in fact it will benefit your arms, wrists and shoulders, as these muscles help support your upper body as you steer the bike and keep it on track.

Joints : Cycling exercises your joints and helps keep them supple. Importantly, it does this in a gentle way. When you sit on a bike about 70 percent of your weight is supported by the saddle, handlebars and pedals. The pedalling motion is smooth and the effort you need to apply can be varied by changing gear which allows you to do more or less work according to how your joints are feeling. Cycling will exercise the muscles around the joints which improves their stability. Blood flow to the joints is enhanced and this helps maintain healthy cartilage.

Lungs : Oxygen is essential for life and you need a plentiful supply. People who are unfit and who take little exercise often have impaired lung function. Cycling makes you breathe more frequently and deeply, and this brings more oxygen into your bloodstream and removes waste carbon dioxide. You'll burn more calories and have higher energy levels. You're actually likely to notice these benefits when you get off the bike; you no longer feel out of breath climbing stairs, for example.

Blood pressure : Cycling can reduce the risk of your developing high blood pressure, or, if you already have the condition, it can help reduce it. A gentle bike ride will cause your blood pressure to rise for a short time, but when you stop it should soon return to normal. The quicker it does this, the fitter you are likely to be.

Heart : That most amazing organ, the heart, is largely muscle and, like the other muscles in your body, cycling will strengthen it, meaning that it pumps blood more efficiently. Cycling can also help stabilise your cholesterol levels and prevent the build-up of fatty deposits in the arteries of your heart, a condition known as atherosclerosis. It occurs as a result of an invasion and accumulation of white blood cells and this can lead to the artery walls stiffening and restricting blood flow with a consequent increase in blood pressure.

Mind : As well as benefitting physical health, cycling can have a positive effect on mental well-being. Your bike is a great stress buster. A ride lets you escape your worries for a while and put things in perspective. The rhythmic pulse of the pedals has a soothing effect, at times it's close to a state of meditation. You return home in a relaxed, more objective, optimistic frame of mind, and you're more likely to enjoy a good night's sleep. Cycling can improve your self-esteem partly due to the natural "high" that comes after exercise. Scientists are unclear as to exactly why this occurs, possibly it's down to chemicals such as endorphins being released into the bloodstream, but it's a well-documented phenomenon. You're also likely to feel better because you know you look better. Improved blood flow brings with it a healthier complexion and smoother skin. Combine these with stronger limbs, better posture and a lower body weight and – wow! – you're looking good.

Improved blood flow to the brain appears to enhance some aspects of cognitive function and your ability to solve problems. This is useful for everyday life, but it may also enable you to make cognitive leaps and boost your creativity. [7] Many writers, musicians, artists, top executives and all kinds of other professionals use exercise to overcome mental blocks and to help them make good decisions. The composer Edward Elgar was an enthusiastic cyclist and some musicologists claim to hear the rolling rhythms and cadences of bicycling in his works. Albert Einstein was another regular on two wheels and it is claimed that e=mc2 came to him while cycling.

Cycling is good for **you** and it's also an opportunity to help others. Every year sponsored bike rides raise millions of pounds for good causes. And you'll be doing your bit for the environment, both locally and globally, every time you swap a car ride for a bike ride. You'll be easing traffic congestion and cutting carbon emissions and generally making your community a nicer place.

Ride a bike and you'll lose weight, ward off ill health, get fit, look better and probably live longer. Who knows? You may even write the odd symphony or come up with a new theory of relativity.

---

[7]   More research is now showing this link, increasingly recorded in research through studies of academic attainment among physically active students compared with those who are less active.

Booth, J. et al. 2014 Associations between objectively measured physical activity and academic attainment in adolescents from a UK cohort. *British Journal of Sports Medicine.* 48(3), pp.265–270.

Shakespeare wrote of the seven ages of man: the infant, the lover, the soldier, the justice, the foolish pantaloon and the toothless old-timer. It's a rather gloomy take on the ageing process but his point is a sound one: people change over time, and different age groups have different needs and abilities.

The constant throughout life, however – this is me talking now, not Shakespeare – is the need to be physically active. Cycling is a great way to meet that need, to keep your weight under control, stay in good shape and lower your risk of disease. Bikes, like people, come in all shapes and sizes, and there are adaptions, accessories and specialist equipment that will enable almost everyone, even people with complex needs, to enjoy a long and active life on two (or more) wheels. So, with apologies to the Bard, here's my take on the seven ages of man – or indeed, woman.

1. Bumps

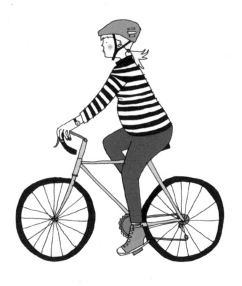

Even the under-zeros can benefit from cycling. Lots of women find it a good way to take gentle exercise during pregnancy and many a bump has been for a bike ride. Cycling can reduce the severity of common problems such as back and pelvic girdle pain, and conditions such as constipation and morning sickness. It can help increase the mother-to be's energy levels and prevent fatigue. It can fortify mental and emotional well-being too by helping to relieve stress, reduce or prevent depression, and promote a good night's sleep.

Many pregnant women have found that cycling helps them cope with the demands of labour and birth. Cycling can increase muscle tone, strength and stamina, all of which make for an easier pregnancy and labour. And mothers who are fit will find it easier get back into shape after the baby is born.

Exercise during pregnancy can be good for the developing child as well as for the mother. There is mounting evidence that babies born to active mums tend to have more robust cardiovascular systems from an early age than those born to mothers who are more sedentary. Exercise may even boost the baby's brain development.[8,9] As with any form of exercise during pregnancy, talk to your GP or midwife if you have any concerns. Cycling should be fine for you as long as you feel safe, confident and comfortable while doing so. Some women pedal right up to their eighth month of pregnancy, some stop sooner. There are no hard and fast rules. Comfort can often be increased by wearing appropriate clothing (see Chapter Five) and by raising the height of your handlebars (see Chapter Four).

2. Babies

New-born babies are allowed a short break from cycling, but after about eight months, once they are able to sit up and hold their heads up unaided, they're ready to see the world from the vantage point of a child seat or cycle trailer. Youngsters usually take to it with alacrity, they like the sensation of movement and respond with gurgles of satisfaction.

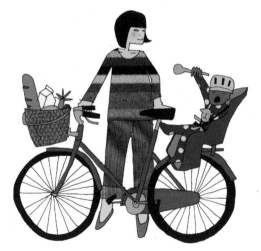

Child seats come in two types. Forward-mounted seats fit on the bike's top tube or crossbar and allow you to keep an eye on your passenger and to talk to them. However, you might find steering the bike difficult with a baby up front, in which case go for the second type, the rear-mounted seat.

Seats that are rated BS EN 14344 are approved to carry children weighing 9–22 kilos.

---

8   American Physiological Society. 2008.
Exercise During Pregnancy Leads To A Healthier Heart In Moms- And Babies-to-be. Science Daily. [Online]. [Accessed 5 January 2015]. Available from: http://www.sciencedaily.com/releases/2008/04/080407114630.htm

9   Labonte-Lemoyne E, Curnier D, Ellemberg D. 2013. *Foetal brain development is influenced by maternal exercise during pregnancy.* (Abstract). Neuroscience 2013 Conference, November 2013, San Diego, California.

Buy from a reputable bike shop and expect to pay at least £40. Spend more and you'll get a seat that reclines (useful for very young children when they want to sleep) and with features such as an adjustable headrest, a rain cover and storage compartments. All seats should have a safety harness and foot guards to keep tiny toes away from the bike's wheels. More information is available from the RoSPA website.

Bike trailers allow you and your offspring to cycle further and take all the paraphernalia of childhood with you. Kids love trailers. They can play with their toys, eat and drink, wave to passers-by, and eventually fall asleep. The child sits on a comfortable hammock-type seat, strapped in with a safety harness and protected further by the trailer's roll-cage. They can enjoy the fresh air on fine days, or be safely tucked away behind wind- and water-proof panels during bad weather.

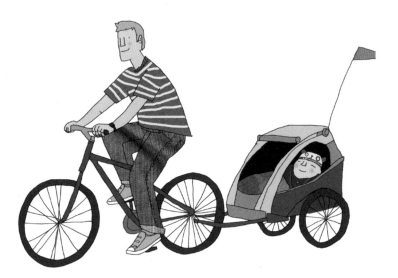

Upmarket trailers convert into stylish baby buggies which can be very handy when you reach your destination. Trailers are considerably more expensive than child seats and you have to get used to the extra weight and width when riding. They were once quite an unusual sight but there are now many brands to choose from. Burley and Chariot are two manufacturers with a lot of experience and a good reputation. There are trailers for a single child and some that will take two.

3. Children

As they get older, children are less content to be mere passengers; they want the fun and the freedom that comes from having a bike of their own. Buy quality kit if you can. Look upon it as an investment in your child's future health and well-being. As we saw in the previous chapter, adults need a minimum of 150 minutes of moderate intensity physical activity every week. Children and young people (ages 5 -18) need at least 60 minutes **every day.** [10] Many get nothing like enough and 19% of children in Year 6 (10-11 year olds) are obese and a further 14.4% are overweight. [11] Sadly, the problem is getting worse rather than better. Capitalise on your child's natural enthusiasm for cycling and there's a good chance they'll maintain the habit, stay at a healthy weight, and grow up to be fit and active adults.

Children can learn to ride a bike as early as three years old and almost all have mastered it by the age of five. Cycling involves a number of skills and a degree of finesse. You can make things easier for your child by breaking the learning process down. First, help them get the hang of balancing on two wheels. Don't bother with stabilisers (two arms either side of the bike with little wheels attached to keep the young rider upright); they're not actually that stable. If the child lurches sharply to one side the stabiliser can act as a pivot and flip the bike over in spectacular fashion. Stabilisers also inhibit the business of learning to balance. A far better way to introduce children to the rudiments of cycling is to use a "balance bike". These devices have two wheels, handlebars and a seat, just like a proper bike, but no pedals or chain. The child sits on it and moves forward by scooting. Kids love the sensation of gliding along under their own power and soon learn to lift their feet up so as to get the most from each scoot. Any problems and they can quickly put both feet to the floor.

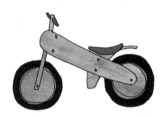

Children as young as two will enjoy playing with a balance bike. When they've fully mastered it, it's time to present them with their first proper bicycle. Do two things: lower the saddle so they can put both feet flat on the ground, and unscrew the

---

10   NHS choices. 2013. *Physical activity guidelines for children and young people.* [Online]. [Accessed 6 January 2015]. Available from: http://www.nhs.uk/Livewell/fitness/Pages/physical-activity-guidelines-for-young-people.aspx

11   2013/14 figures. Public Health England. 2015. *Child obesity.* [Online]. [Accessed 5 January 2015]. Available from: http://www.noo.org.uk/NOO_about_obesity/child_obesity

pedals. Let them scoot along, just as they did on their balance bike. Once they're scooting with confidence they can get to grips with the basics of steering and braking. Mission accomplished, refit the pedals and raise the saddle a little. They'll still be wobbly and unpredictable for a while – but they'll be riding.

Try a tag-along

While your child is learning to ride they're limited to cycling in the garden or on traffic free paths. If you want to venture further afield for a family bike ride try a tag-along or trailer bike. These are child-size bicycles with a tow bar instead of a front wheel. A hinged attachment links it to the adult rider's seatpost and the two of you ride in tandem.

You remain in full control of the steering and braking but both riders pedal – or the rear rider freewheels if they are getting tired. Tag-alongs allow a parent and child to cycle safely in town as well as in open country. Children feel very involved and grown up and adults can relax knowing that Junior isn't riding erratically or pedalling off in the wrong direction.

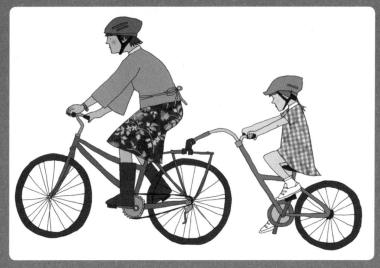

Upmarket tag-alongs have gears so that the youngster can vary their pedalling cadence. Children are ready for a tag-along at about four years old. As they grow, the height of the saddle and the handlebars can be raised. When the tag-along is no longer needed, sell it – they command good prices second-hand.

Many kids' bikes are heavy, poorly made and fitted with flimsy components that are impossible to repair or adjust. On top of that, many parents make the mistake of buying their youngster a bike that is several sizes too large on the assumption that they will grow into it. Don't fall into that trap. Your child will be safer and will learn more rapidly on a decent bike that fits them properly. High-quality children's bicycles take some tracking down and you'll pay at least twice what you would for a bike from a supermarket or toy store, but it's well worth the extra expense. The bikes are little gems: lightweight and well equipped, specially proportioned to fit small riders and to give them a taste of real cycling. Islabikes, Frog Bikes and Puky are respected brands.

When your child can balance, steer, and brake and is capable of taking one hand off the handlebars and look behind them without too much wobbling they're ready for Bikeability training. Bikeability is the new updated version of the classic Cycling Proficiency Test. The instructors are experienced cyclists and the courses have to meet a consistent standard. Bikeability aims to equip young people (and adults too: see Chapter Six) with the knowledge, skills and confidence to carry out proper journeys. Find out whether your local council's road safety team offers Bikeability training. Check too whether there are any independent training providers in your area. These small, community-minded organisations are passionate about cycling and they employ dedicated people with a vast knowledge and expertise.

Bikeability

Bikeability training has three levels with badges, booklets and certificates are awarded for passing each level:

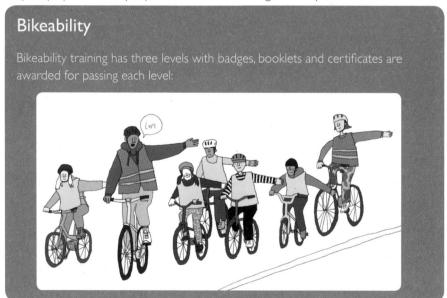

- **Level One** (red badge) is a beginners' course that teaches children how to control their bikes properly and to carry out basic manoeuvres. It takes place off-road, away from traffic.

- **Level Two** (amber badge) introduces children to riding on the road. They learn how to start and stop, pull out of junctions, turn left and right and pass parked cars.

- **Level Three** (green badge) is the advanced course. It teaches young cyclists how to use roundabouts and multi-lane roads, and how to negotiate complex junctions.

4. Teens

As they grow children become more independently minded. They want to go off on their own, meet their friends, make their own way to school or college. Cycling should be exactly right for them: a cheap, customisable, highly individual form of travel that's available 24/7.

Parents sometimes worry because there are risks associated with putting an impetuous inexperienced youngster on a bike and letting them out on their own. Risk, however, needs to be put in perspective: cycling is actually a surprisingly safe mode of transport and the health benefits (we looked at these in Chapter One) substantially outweigh the dangers. It tends to be the couch potatoes, not the regular cyclists, who pile on the pounds and who go on to develop heart disease, diabetes or other chronic conditions. [12]

Cycling can be made safer if your child has completed their Bikeability training. If they've received training at school make sure that they've gone all the way through to Bikeability Level 3. This is the part of the training that covers riding in a range of traffic conditions on real-life roads. Trainees learn how to develop their control skills, judge speed and distance, plan a route, and to negotiate complex junctions, roundabouts, multi-lane roads and traffic lights.

If your teenager has not yet achieved Level 3 book them onto a course. If they're

---

12   British Medical Association. 1992. *Cycling: Towards Health and Safety.* Oxford: Oxford University Press.

resistant to being trained in a group environment book them a series of one-to-one lessons. Many cycle training providers offer a choice of male or female trainers. Matching your son or daughter to a trainer of the same sex sometimes makes it more palatable for them. They might also like the idea of getting their hands dirty and going on a bike maintenance course. If you know that your child can put their chain back on, keep their brakes working and cope with a puncture it gives everyone peace of mind.

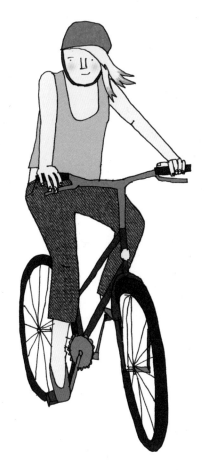

I've known parents make a little contract with their teenage kids. Yes, we'll buy you that bike you're pestering us for. Yes, you can go off on your own and meet your mates; but in return you complete your Bikeability training, you wear a helmet and hi-vis, you use lights after dark, you lock the bike up properly, and you text us an OK message as soon as you arrive at your destination. This is wise parenting. It's giving kids some of the freedom they crave but it's also showing them that with freedom comes responsibility. Most teenagers rise to the challenge and fulfil their part of the deal.

Some parents find they have the opposite problem. Far from being eager to cycle, their teenagers seem to lose all interest. Young people can be very unpredictable; the vagaries of fashion and the opinions of their peers may radically affect their choices. They may come to regard cycling as hideously uncool. If, despite your best endeavours, your child appears to give up on cycling, don't despair, and there's little point in nagging them. Some people lapse for years, decades even, until something tempts them back onto the bike.

Five tips for teen management

- **Bike :** Buy a mid-range model. Your son or daughter may aspire to a top-of-the range bike, but an expensive machine is much more likely to be stolen. On the other hand a really cheap bike has no cachet and will be unreliable.

- **Clothes :** Teenagers can be incredibly style conscious and are unlikely to appreciate being kitted out in a hi-vis tabard with matching arm- or leg-bands. Happily, there's plenty of gear out there that's likely to meet with their approval including tops that are grungy by day but bright at night. Or, if that's not an option, you may find they'll accept a backpack with reflective trim. Make certain that their bike has the required reflectors (see Chapter Four) and encourage them to pimp their ride with reflective strips or transfers.

- **Helmet :** Many parents want their child to wear a cycle helmet; many kids are reluctant to do so. If you force the issue the risk is that the child simply pedals off wearing the helmet and then removes it once they round the first corner. The trick is to make helmet wearing appear natural, normal and, if possible, to give it a degree of street cred. The manufacturers have helped by producing a huge range of styles and colours. Let your child choose a designer model rather than impose a supermarket special on them. Or try gently steering your child's attention to role models in the world of BMX and road racing. If Danny MacGaskill or Bradley Wiggins wears a helmet, maybe they'll want to as well. There's more about cycle helmets in Chapter Five.

- **Lights :** Teenagers can be absent-minded. If they're likely to forget their lights then consider fitting lights that stay attached to the bike. There are various brands of lockable light available. Or try Pedalites. The clue is in the name: the lights are powered by a tiny generator within the body of the pedal which means that there are no batteries or switches to worry about. The act of pedalling charges them up and after a few minutes riding the lights will stay on even when the bike is stationary. They're not a substitute for proper front and rear lights, but they're a great addition – bright, maintenance free, always there.

- **Lock :** Buy a good quality lock (see Chapter Four). It will have at least two keys. Give one to your son or daughter; keep the spares somewhere safe in case key number one goes missing. Retain the instructions that come with the lock: they will tell you how to order replacement keys if (OK, when) all the original ones have been lost.

5. Young adults

Many young people rediscover cycling when they go to university, others when they get their first job and need wheels for work. This is when the advantages of the bike as a form of transport become clear. A bike is reliable, easy to park and for short rush-hour journeys it can be the fastest vehicle across town. There's no time wasted in traffic queues or the misery of standing on the bus or tube with your face in someone's armpit. For many students and young workers money is tight and here cycling really scores. The cost of bus or train fares can make a serious dent in a new worker's wage packet, while buying and running a car or even a moped may be entirely out of reach. But a bicycle, at a fraction of the cost, can pretty much match the car's flexibility. You travel at a time that suits you, day or night, making it ideal for shift workers or people on flexible contracts.

There's mounting evidence that cyclists are more productive at the workplace: they arrive on time, alert and ready for action, they're less stressed and less likely to take time off due to illness. [13] It's not so well known that cycling can also increase your brain power. A paper published in the British Journal of Sports Medicine found that a mere 5% improvement in fitness from cycling led to an improvement of up to 15% in mental capacity by stimulating cell regeneration in the area of the hippocampus, the part of the brain responsible for memory and spatial awareness. The hippocampus typically starts to degrade around age 30 and cycling can have a massive impact in reducing this deterioration. [14]

Cycling can also make you more creative. Just 25 minutes of aerobic exercise improves the flow of oxygen to the brain. This sparks your inactive neurons into life, allowing your brain to handle its workload more efficiently and helping you to be more creative with your problem solving.

Cycling to work will help you prepare you for the day ahead, and cycling home will help you unwind and recover from the day you've just had. You'll sleep well, be less stressed, your immune system will be boosted and you'll look good. [15]

13   2014. The Telegraph. 2013. *Cycling 'halves the number of sick days' taken by staff.* [Online]. [Accessed 5 January 2015]. Available from: http://www.telegraph.co.uk/men/active/recreational-cycling/10097449/Cycling-halves-the-number-of-sick-days-taken-by-staff.html

14   Kirk I. Erickson et al. 2011. Exercise training increases size of hippocampus and improves memory. Proceedings of the National Academy of Sciences 108(7), pp.3017–3022

15   University of East Anglia. 2014. *Walking or cycling to work improves wellbeing, University of East Anglia researchers find.* [Online]. [Accessed 5 January 2015]. Available from: https://www.uea.ac.uk/mac/comm/media/press/2014/september/active-commuting-benefits

Increased circulation through exercise delivers oxygen and nutrients to skin cells more effectively, while flushing harmful toxins out. Exercise also creates an ideal environment within the body to optimise collagen production, helping reduce the appearance of wrinkles and speed up the healing process.[16] Astute bosses are bound to notice this fresh-faced young dynamo as they stride into work each morning, and rapid promotion is sure to follow!

6. Mature adults

Middle-aged people, particularly women, gain weight more easily. Between the ages of 30 and 40 changes to the metabolism lead to the laying down of fat. Brown fat, the so-called "good" fat, which is present in all of us at birth, steadily declines and by the time we are middle-aged it is replaced by white fat, the "bad" visceral fat which clings to hips to waistlines: the notorious "middle-age spread".[17]

At the same time as gaining fat tissue, our heart rate increases and the proportion of muscle in our bodies begins to decrease, both of which slow down our metabolism. Our energy needs drop because fat tissue requires less energy (in the form of calories) to maintain its functions compared with muscle. If you're burning fewer calories but haven't changed your diet you're going to gain weight.

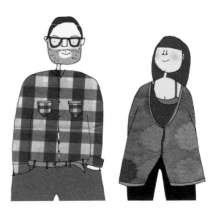

Meanwhile, our production of growth hormone decreases. This is the hormone that is vital for muscle, bone and tendon strength, for exercise efficiency and injury prevention, as well as making your body use fat reserves as a primary fuel source. The consequences can be lower back, neck or shoulder pains, trapped nerves and headaches. With women in particular, the reduction in peak bone mass accelerates from their 50's onwards because of hormonal changes linked to the menopause,

---

16   Employees who cycle regularly to work are less frequently ill, with on average more than one day per year less absenteeism than colleagues who do not cycle to work.
    2014. TNO Knowledge for business. 2009. *Reduced sickness absence in regular commuter cyclists can save employers 27 million euros.* [Online]. [Accessed 5 January 2015].
Available from: http://www.vcl.li/bilder/518.pdf Employees who cycle regularly to work are less frequently ill, with on average more than one day per year less absenteeism than colleagues who do not cycle to work.

17   Visceral fat is the fat embedded around the liver and other internal organs. It has a powerful pro-inflammatory effect and is closely related to obesity.

making osteoporosis a major concern. This leaves joints and bones susceptible to overuse and misuse injury.

These natural processes are compounded further by lifestyle factors. Middle-age, for many, is a time when their incomes are relatively high. At work their role is more likely to be desk-based than physically active. They can afford good food and drink, a reliable car, and a houseful of labour saving gadgets. The consequence is a decline in the amount of exercise they take – at the very time when it would be particularly beneficial. Regular physical activity, as we saw in Chapter One, can help relieve aches and pains, prevent weight gain, and head off serious health problems.

Cycle to work and live longer

Amongst many health professionals the Copenhagen Heart Study[18] is famous. The study followed the health of 13,375 women and 17,265 men aged between 20-93 years over a period of 14 years. Of these 15,000 cycled regularly, including 7,000 who cycled to work. The research shows that cycling to work decreased the overall risk of death (including risk of accidents). The authors state that "even after adjustment for other risk factors, including leisure time physical activity, those who did not cycle to work experienced a 39% higher mortality rate than those who did".

By all means enjoy the trappings of success, but don't neglect the bike. Cycling isn't just for the apprentice or the office junior, it's ideal for managers and executives too. All kinds of very successful people ride bikes. Famous names include the tycoon Sir Alan Sugar, architect Sir Norman Foster, fashion designers Paul Smith and Jeff Banks, comedian Dave Gorman, actor Alistair McGowan, broadcasters Jeremy Paxman, Andrew Neil and Jon Snow, songsters Madonna, Lady Gaga and Lily Allen... it's a long list. In business circles cycling has been dubbed the "new golf." Executives are using bike rides in the same way that they'd previously used a round on the golf links – to have fun, keep fit, develop their networks of contacts and cut deals.

7. Seniors

There's really no age at which cycling stops being an option. As you get older cycling can be a key part of an active and enjoyable retirement, helping you maintain fitness

---

18   Andersen, L., Schnohr, P., Schroll, M. and Hein, H. 2000. All-cause mortality associated with physical activity during leisure time, work, sports, and cycling to work. *Archives of Internal Medicine*. 160, pp. 1621-1628.

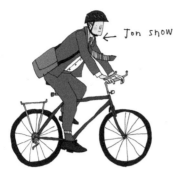

Jon snow

and keeping you engaged with the wider world. Take a trip to the Netherlands and you'll immediately notice the number of silver-haired cyclists. Over there, people aged 65 or more make nearly one-in-four of their trips by bike.

As you age you may prefer a bike built for comfort rather than speed. A more upright riding position will relieve pressure on your wrists, hands and back, a frame without a top-tube or crossbar will be easier to get on and off. Electric assistance can also be beneficial, ironing out the hills, shrinking distances and making it possible to carry even heavy loads with little effort. You might even choose to swap two wheels for the stately stability of a tricycle. That's what happened to Octavio Orduño of Long Beach, California. He gave up riding his bicycle at the age of 100 – mainly at the insistence of his wife. Instead, he began using a tricycle for the daily ride round his neighbourhood. He was still going strong at 103.

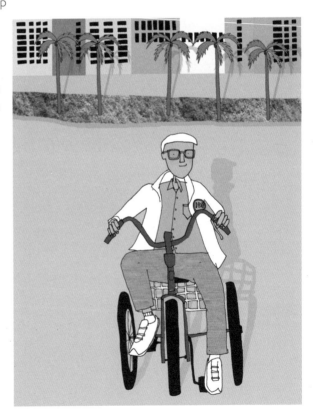

The bike

Every cyclist needs a bike! A comfortable bike that fits you properly is a joy to use – and it's likely to be used. On the other hand, an unwieldy lump of a machine with a rock-hard saddle will be relegated to the shed after a few weeks. This chapter is about buying a bike, or if you already have one, preparing it for the road.

Let's begin by looking at the different types of bike. There's a breathtaking range of bikes to choose from, each made for a specific purpose. To the uninitiated they all look pretty similar but there are significant differences between them. Here are some of the principal types:

Mountain bikes are the rugged 4x4s of the cycling world. They come with front, and often rear, suspension, knobbly tyres, powerful brakes and numerous gears. The handlebars are wide and straight for maximum control. Mountain bikes are designed for off-road use: on tarmac they can feel sluggish compared with lighter bikes. 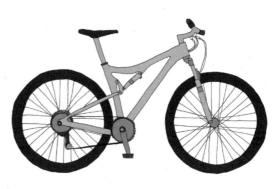 Nevertheless, many people find the upright riding position, hill climbing ability and go-anywhere, do-anything nature of a mountain bike ideal for urban terrain too.

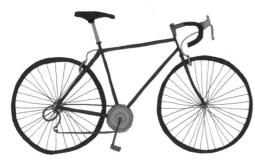 **Road bikes**, or racing bikes, are cycling's greyhounds. Think Tour de France, think Lycra. The ride can be on the harsh side and you may find the dropped-down, aerodynamic riding position uncomfortable. Road bikes are delicate creatures, easily damaged if you charge through potholes or off a kerb. On the plus side though, the minimalist construction, ultra-light weight and skinny tyres makes for speed, responsiveness and an exhilaration that's relished by enthusiasts of all ages.

Hybrids, or trekking bikes, combine the multi-geared toughness of a mountain bike with a little of the agility and lightness of a road bike. They're likely to come equipped with mudguards (maybe a chainguard as well) and a luggage rack. The tyres are smooth in the middle for road riding with knobbly edges for off-road grip. Hybrid bikes are good all-rounders, fine in town but equally at home on forest trails and cycle tracks.

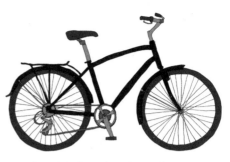

City bikes, sometimes called comfort bikes, are intended for sedate urban cycling over relatively short distances. They're likely to have an open, step-through frame and an upright riding position. Gears are housed inside the rear wheel hub. Mudguards and a chainguard help keep you and the bike clean. Expect a luggage rack at the back, a soft saddle in the middle and quite possibly a basket at the front.

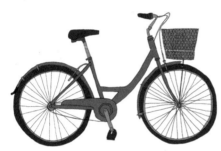

Touring bikes, or expedition bikes, are cycling's mile-eaters. There's some resemblance to a road bike, but a tourer is many times stronger and much more comfortable whether you're tootling up the High Street or exploring the Great Silk Road. Some have straight handlebars; some have dropped bars that allow you to hold on in different positions, reducing fatigue over long distances. You get lots of equipment on a tourer: gears galore, strong racks for panniers, tough mudguards, cages to hold water bottles and a comfy saddle.

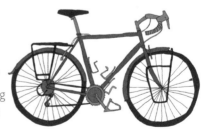

Folding bikes are relatively expensive and their small wheels and strangely shaped frames can mean a twitchy ride. Hills can be a struggle and they don't cover distances as effortlessly as big-wheeled bikes. That said, folders have many advantages. They make it possible to combine a car, train, boat or plane journey

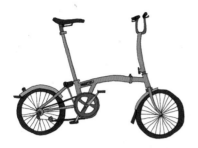

with a bike ride, and when you reach your destination the bike can be collapsed and stowed away in a small space where you can keep an eye on it. For city dwellers, day trippers and commuters a folding bike is well worth considering.

Electric bikes, or e-bikes, are big business in the far-east and a common site on the streets and cycle tracks of most northern European countries. They're gradually becoming more popular in the UK. There are the "twist and go" type where you turn a switch on the handlebar grip to trigger electric assistance, and the more sophisticated "pedelec" type, where sensors detect the effort that you're putting in via the pedals and then add a bit of boost.

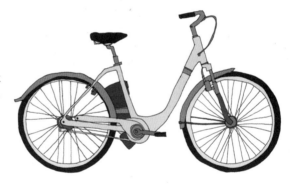

There are numerous brands of electric bike available, some are of very dubious quality. Research the market before you buy. You want to be confident that the dealer who sells you the bike will still be trading when back-up is required. Look into battery replacement too. Good quality batteries can be charged and depleted numerous times, nasty ones can fail to recharge properly after less than a year's use and a replacement can be very expensive. The better dealers offer a guaranteed number of charges and a promise of a replacement if the battery fails.

If you're taking up cycling to get fit it may seem counterintuitive to go for an electric bike. In fact, you're still getting all the benefits of gentle exercise, the bike merely adds a bit of assistance. Furthermore, many enthusiasts find themselves using their e-bike for errands and shopping trips they would otherwise do by car, a substitution that's good for both the rider and the environment.

Whatever type of bike you go for set yourself a realistic budget. For about £150 you'll get a basic, no-frills bike. It may possibly have mudguards and a luggage rack. If not, these items and any other accessories will all cost extra. So, be prepared to pay at least £200 for the total package. Spend more if you possibly can – think of it as an investment. £500 will buy you a bike that's noticeably lighter and with better-quality components. It'll be easier to ride, more reliable and last longer.

You might be able to get your employer to help with the purchase if they're signed up to the Government's Cycle to Work Scheme. The scheme gives employers generous tax breaks that allow them to purchase bikes and sell them on to their staff, deducting a small amount from the employee's pay packet each month. Savings depend on the nature of the business and the employee's tax band, but it's possible to get a bike plus accessories for almost half price. See if your employer runs such a scheme and, if they don't, suggest that they start.

Evaluate as many different bikes as you can by reading reviews and road tests on-line and in bike magazines, and pick the brains of any real-life cyclists you happen to know. Start visiting bike shops. Even in the age of chain stores, on-line retailers and mail-order operations the High Street bike shop is going strong. These businesses survive, indeed thrive, because they know their job. A bike from a proper cycle shop will cost you more than one from a cheapo outlet, but you will be buying a better product, plus, at no extra charge, precious expertise and support.

Once you're beyond merely browsing, ask to take two or three bikes for a test ride. Good cycle shops will encourage you to do this, although they may not have the bikes all set up and ready to ride, in which case your road tests will have to be scheduled for another day. The shop will also want some guarantee that you and the bike are going to reappear, so they'll ask for ID and a deposit. A credit card swipe is usually sufficient.

Take the bike somewhere quiet and get a feel for how it fits, rides and responds. Are the handlebars the right height and shape? Does the bike corner easily? Is the ride smooth or sharp? Are the brakes soft or fierce? Do the gears change smoothly? (Though bear in mind that gear changing requires a light touch – duff changes might be down to you, rather than the bike). Even a short ride will reveal important differences and help you to make a more informed choice.

If you're on a tight budget and a new bike is beyond your reach, go for a second-hand model. Websites such as eBay, Gum Tree, Craigslist, Freecycle and cycle specialists such as Going Going Bike have great potential – if you know what you're looking for. There are several points in their favour. You get to see pictures of the advertised bike and there's a much fuller description than in a newspaper or magazine advert. You can usually e-mail questions to the seller or forward the ad to knowledgeable friends for their opinion. The downside is that you're not able to try the bike or examine it thoroughly before buying it. You might end up with a "bargain" that requires an extensive – and expensive – round of repairs before it's rideable. Ex-hire bikes are worth considering too. In the autumn and winter many rental businesses sell off some of their older bikes (although "older" is a relative term: it might only mean last year's model) and there are often deals to be made. The bikes may be a bit scuffed and scratched, but hire centres tend to run strong, reliable machines and they will have been well maintained. Find a hire business and chat up the proprietor.

Eventually, your research and road tests lead you to a decision point. There's a bike you rather like and there's a sum of money to be handed over. Two-, three-, five-hundred pounds; maybe a lot more. A slight feeling of panic is understandable. Relax and pay up with a smile. Compared with life's other major purchases, bicycles are unbeatable value. A bike will provide endless enjoyment, it will help keep you slim and healthy, and if you use it for day-to-day transport it will return your investment in less than a year.

If you buy a new bike it **should** have received a PDI (a pre-delivery inspection) and be set up correctly with everything working properly. But even the best bike shops sometimes miss something, so it's advisable to inspect the bike yourself. If you buy a second-hand bike, or if you dig out an old machine that's been hibernating at the back of the garage or tucked away in the garden shed, it's most unlikely to be in perfect condition and will definitely benefit from being checked over.

Anyone can perform a bike check. It simply means looking carefully and closely at every part of the bike and trying to spot any wear or damage. The diagram over the page shows a typical bike and names its various parts.

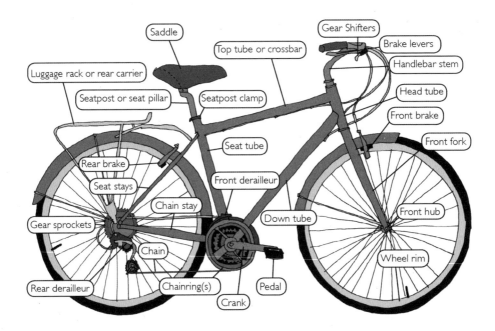

Cycle training instructors who sometimes have to check dozens of bikes at a time for roadworthiness have brought a bit of method to the process. They call it the M-shaped check. You can also do it with the bike turned upside down, at which point it becomes the W-shaped check! This is what you do:

- Start with the **front wheel hub.** The quick-release fastening or wheel nuts should be tight. The wheel should spin freely with no wobbling and no more than a few millimetres of side-to-side movement.
- Check for missing or loose **spokes.** When you pluck them they should make a musical twang. The **front tyre** should be pumped up hard. Check it for signs of wear or cracks and splits. Remove any debris that might be stuck in the tread.
- Spin the front wheel and apply the **brake.** It should stop the wheel almost instantly and prevent it turning. Check the **brake pads** for signs of wear and ensure that they grip the wheel rim but don't touch the tyre. The brake cable shouldn't be frayed.
- The **handlebars** should turn smoothly and the handlebar stem needs to be aligned with the front fork. The stem shouldn't be raised beyond the maximum extension mark. Inspect the **frame** for signs of rust or damage.

- The **pedals** should spin freely and be attached tightly to the **cranks.** The cranks themselves should be fastened firmly to the **bottom bracket** with no more than a smidgeon of side-to-side movement.
- Check that the teeth of the **chainring** are not worn and, if there is more than one chainring, ensure that that the chain will shift easily between rings. The cable should not be frayed. Check that the **chain** is lightly oiled and that, when you change gear, it moves freely from **sprocket** to **sprocket**. Look out for corroded or damaged chain links.
- The **seatpost** should be set at the correct height (never beyond its maximum extension mark) and secured tightly. The **saddle** should be firmly attached.
- The **back brake**, its **cable, wheel, tyre** and **hub** should be checked in the same way as those at the front. The **gears** should shift easily. The cable should be intact with no fraying. The **derailleur** should be clean and undamaged. If the bike has a rear **luggage rack** or **mudguards** ensure that all the fastenings are tight and that no part of the rack or mudguard rubs against the tyre.

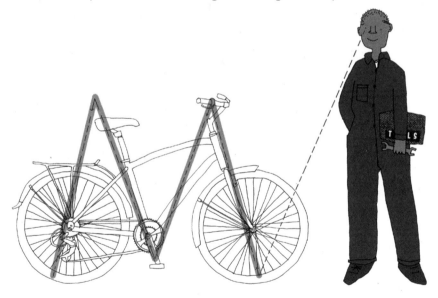

If this all sounds a bit overwhelming, book the bike in for a service at your local cycle shop. A mechanic will check everything and adjust your gears and brakes, replace worn cables and brake blocks, and lubricate the parts that need it. They'll tell you about any underlying problems likely to need attention in the near future.

Comfort **4**

Some people think that comfort and cycling can't possibly go together. That's simply not true. If you're new to cycling, or returning to it after a gap of several years, it may take a while to get used to balancing, pedalling, steering and moving up and down the gears while perched on a saddle. The trick is to ease yourself into it gently and to remember that cycling shouldn't hurt. You may find it hard work at first and your nether regions may feel a little tender – but that's not the same as pain.

Make sure that your bike is the correct size and that it's set it up properly. Just about everything on a bike can be adjusted or swapped for something better. Whatever your shape, size or riding style, with perseverance and patience you can achieve a perfect fit. Eventually, hopping on your bike will feel as natural and as comfortable as slipping into a well-worn pair of walking shoes.

With the exception of most folding bikes, which come in a one-size-fits-all format, bike manufacturers offer a range of frame sizes. Buy a bike that's too small and you'll be squashed up with bits of you colliding with bits of the bike. Buy one that's too big and you won't be able to control the thing properly. Straddle the bike of your choice and stand with both feet flat on the floor. There should be at least an inch (25mm) of clearance between your crotch and the top tube or crossbar. You'll want more clearance if it's a mountain bike and you plan to go bounding about off-road.

With someone holding the bike upright, sit on the saddle and place the ball of each foot (that's the part just behind your toes) on the pedals. Pedal backwards slowly. When your foot is at the bottom of the pedal stroke your knee should be slightly bent. You should also be able to slide off the saddle and put both feet to the floor. Do some more reverse pedalling and now try squeezing the brakes and reaching for the gear controls. You may have to lean forward slightly, but you shouldn't have to stretch.

As well as coming in different sizes, bikes are often made gender-specific. Women generally have slightly shorter arms and torsos than men, and female bike frames are proportioned accordingly making them more comfortable for women to ride.

Women's bikes often have a sloping crossbar or top tube, on the basis that such a design will be more decorous to ride when wearing a flowing skirt. The drawback is that "open" frames of this kind tend to be weaker and heavier than conventional

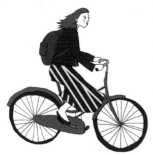

frames so many women opt for a closed or "man's" frame. Equally, many mature gentlemen find that it's a struggle to mount a bike with a crossbar, so they go for an open frame. This is the 21st century. Let's end the man's bike / woman's bike distinction. Just buy the sort that feels most comfortable.

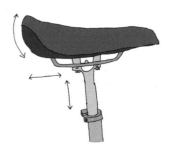

Once you start using your new bike you're likely to discover that the fit falls just short of perfection. That's easily sorted with a few adjustments and replacements. Here are three simple adjustments:

Saddle. Your saddle has a surprising degree of adjustment potential. Set it to what feels like the right position and then go for a short ride, stopping to make further finer adjustments as necessary.

- **Height.** Pull the quick-release lever open, or slacken off the seatpost bolt. Move the post up or down. Take care not to exceed the maximum extension mark.
- **Reach.** Release the bolt underneath the saddle to slide it back or forward.
- **Tilt.** You can even adjust the slope of the saddle slightly if you wish.

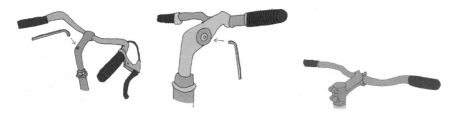

Handlebars. Your comfort may be improved by altering the height of your handlebars. Bars set too low can mean aching arms and a stiff neck. Too high can also be uncomfortable and it may impair your control of the bike.

- **Headset Allen bolt.** Undo this to move your handlebars up or down by a couple of inches. Take care not to exceed the maximum extension mark.
- **Variable stem.** Often fitted to city bikes and hybrids, this is easily adjustable with an Allen key.
- **Threadless headset** (often branded as "Aheadset"). Bikes with this sort of

handlebar mounting can't be adjusted easily. However, if you need more height or reach, it's possible to substitute a longer or shorter stem or one that holds the bars at a different angle. Your bike shop will be able to advise you.

Brakes. It should be easy to reach and operate your bike's brakes.

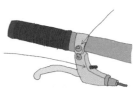

- **Brake mounting bolt.** Loosen the bolt and twist the brake units round the bars to a position where you can reach them easily. Tighten the bolt.
- **Setscrew.** Turn the tiny screw on the inside of the brake unit clockwise to move the brake levers nearer to you.

When you buy a TV or a laptop or a dishwasher, you are buying an integrated unit and you have to take what you are given; but with a bicycle you're in control. If any component meets with your displeasure you can usually swap it for something better. Even simple changes will alter the bike's feel and performance considerably. Here are three easy replacements:

Saddle. Bike makers know that saddles are a matter of personal choice and many fit a cheap, foam-filled saddle as standard, expecting you to replace it. There are various types you may wish to try.

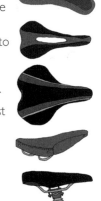

- **Racing.** Firm and narrow. Tends to suit lithe, lightweight riders.
- **Mattress.** Springs underneath cushion the bumps.
- **Gel-filled.** The gel squidges itself to the shape of your bottom.
- **Holey.** The gap is meant to provide a little ventilation and ease the pressure on your more delicate parts.
- **Gender-specific.** Saddles designed for the female form tend to be wider and shorter than those made for men.
- **Classic leather.** The high-quality hide gradually softens and conforms to the shape of your nether regions, rather as a pair of handmade shoes fits your feet. Brooks is probably the most famous manufacturer of leather saddles.
- You might also consider a **suspension seatpost** for extra springiness. It telescopes up and down by a few centimetres, ironing out the jolts.

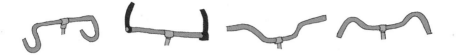

Handlebars. Bikes often come with straight bars set low down. They look very sporty but they force you to adopt a stretched-out riding position which many people find uncomfortable. You might prefer bars of a different shape.

- **Riser bars.** Allow you to ride in a more upright position.
- **Curved bars.** Ease the pressure on your wrists.
- **Dropped bars.** An acquired taste, but the first choice for racers and many long-distance cyclists.
- **Bar ends.** Can be attached to most handlebar types. They enable you to move your hands into slightly different positions as you ride and so avoid numbness. Some bar ends are bare metal, some are ergonomically shaped and padded to support you hands.
- **Grips.** The two bits of the handlebars where you place your hands can be replaced. Ergonomically-shaped gel- or foam-filled grips are more comfortable to hold and provide extra cushioning for your hands.

Tyres. The handlebars and the saddle are two points where bike and body converge. The tyres are the point where the whole caboodle meets the road and they have a crucial effect on the way the bike handles and rides. There are several types:

- **Knobbly.** Fine for mountains and mud, but on tarmac they provide little grip and take more effort to move.
- **Slick.** A smooth tyre with recessed tread. Provides good grip and an easy ride on dry tarmac roads.
- **Semi-slick.** Meant to give you the best of both worlds. A slick tyre with knobbly bits at the edges for when you ride off road.

The inner-tubes inside your tyres gradually lose air. It's hard work riding on a soft tyre and they're more prone to wear and to punctures. If your tyres are really squashy you risk damaging the wheel. Buy a **pump** and practise using it. There are mini-pumps, which can be carried in a bike bag or pocket and longer ones that fasten to the bike. Pumps described as "double action" deliver a blast of air into the tyre when they're pulled as well as pushed, so they're twice as effective. Track pumps (sometimes called floor pumps) are for home or workshop use. They stand upright and you use both hands to push a T-shaped handle. Many cyclists carry a mini-pump for emergencies and keep a track pump back at base for serious inflation.

Check that the business end of your pump fits on to your inner tubes' valves. There are two types of valve in common use: a thick one (called car type or Schrader) and a thin one (called Presta). Some pumps fit only the one sort, some fit both. You can buy adaptors if you have a mismatch.

While you're in maintenance mode, have a look at your **chain** too. A healthy chain is shiny and it glides along almost silently. If it's dry and noisy or even (horror!) showing signs of rust it makes pedalling hard work. Apply oil immediately. There are many different types available. I'm rather fond of the Green Oil brand because of the company's environmental credentials but any oil is better than none. Prop the bike upright, hold a pedal, rotate the crank backwards and dribble a drop or two of oil onto each link of the chain. Do this for a complete revolution of the entire chain until every bit is covered. Then hold an old rag round it and turn the chain backwards again. Use the rag to soak up the surplus oil and to work the remainder into each link. If any oil has sprayed onto your wheel rims or brake pads wipe it off.

Your comfort will be boosted further if you let your bike carry your luggage for you. The alternatives; a rucksack, shoulder bag or pockets filled to bursting point, makes for a less stable ride and the possibility of backache. It's surprising, the amount of stuff you carry on a bike: tools, maps, items of clothing, phone, camera, food and drink, wallet or purse, to say nothing of any items bought en route.

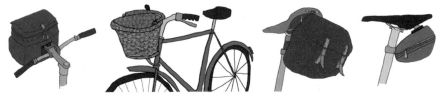

Luggage can be carried on the front of the bike in a handlebar bag or basket, and on the back in a bag that attaches to your saddle or seatpost. Many bikes come with a luggage rack or "rear carrier" as standard. If your bike hasn't got one it's usually easy to fit one. Luggage can then be lashed to the rack using stretchy lengths of elastic with hooks either end that cyclists call bungee straps. They're available from most bike shops and hardware stores.

Racks also take up to two panniers, one either side. These
are bags made specifically for cycling. They distribute the load
evenly and carry it close to the ground (rather than up high as
with a rucksack), giving your bike a lower centre of gravity and
making it more stable. A single pannier is usually enough for
commuting and short leisure rides. A bulkier load will require a
pair.

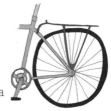

Panniers come in various sizes – the
largest are able to swallow an impressive
50 litres' worth of luggage per pannier.
Some designs are just a simple bag,
others have useful side pockets for
storing smaller items. The better panniers
from companies such as Ortlieb, Altura
and Carradice have nifty fastening
mechanisms that let you attach them and
unclip them in seconds but which won't
shake loose accidentally.

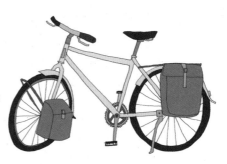

Now for two final accessories. These won't add to your physical comfort, but they
will give you great peace of mind. Firstly, a **lock**. Thousands and thousands of bikes
are stolen every year and most are never reunited
with their owners. All bikes are at risk so you
need to invest in a quality lock. The classic bike
lock is D-shaped. The best ones from companies
such as Kryptonite, Squire, Abus and Trelock have
sophisticated mechanisms and are made from
specially hardened steel. Open the lock and it splits
into two pieces. The curved bar goes through the
bike's frame, through one of the wheels and then
around an immovable object such as a bike stand. You then fit the two bits together
and turn the key to lock it. It takes just a few seconds and quickly becomes second
nature.

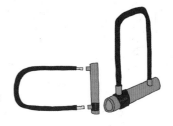

For extra security you can thread a length of cable with loops either end through the
bike's other wheel, through the rails under your saddle, and through anything else that
might be stolen. Secure the loops within the bar of the D-lock.

Be prepared to spend about 10 percent of the cost of your bike on a lock. Those with a **Sold Secure logo** on the packaging have been through an accreditation process that includes trying to force, cut and pick the lock. They are awarded a bronze, silver or gold accolade according to how well they withstand the assault. Go for gold if you can afford it.

ParkThatBike

I despise bike thieves and a couple of years ago I resolved to try and do something to improve the nation's cycle parking. The result is www.ParkThatBike.info a website that lets you do two things.

Firstly, you can ask for cycle parking to be installed. If your local library, station or swimming pool has nowhere to secure a bike, or if there's a road or street that would benefit from a few bike stands simply go to www.ParkThatBike.info and make the request.

Secondly, the website lets you report cycle parking that's damaged, out-dated or badly designed and to ask for proper Sheffield stands to be installed. There are still thousands rusty racks and other horrible forms of bike parking out there. Let's get them ripped out and replaced with something better.

The site uses Google mapping to let you mark the location precisely and you can upload photographs if you wish. You can comment on cycle parking on the public highway, in public spaces, and at busy destinations such as leisure centres, shopping malls and surgeries. All comments are sent to the relevant local authority so that they can take action. It's quick and easy to use – and your ideas make a real difference.

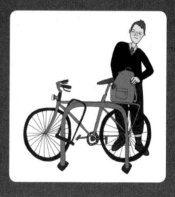

The final accessory to think about is lighting. New bikes should be fitted with a clear white reflector at the front and a red one at the back. There should also be white or yellow reflectors on each wheel (or sometimes the tyres will have a reflective strip on them) and little yellow reflectors on the front and back of each pedal. Reflectors are a legal requirement, although many retailers don't appear to realise this, so your bike may not have them. And consider yourself truly blessed if your new bike comes equipped with lights. You'll almost certainly need to add them. Yes, I realise that you're not planning to ride in the dark but it's surprisingly easy to get caught out. At night (and in the winter months "night" may be 4.00 p.m. in many parts of the UK) the law demands that you use a clear white light at the front and a red one at the rear. Modern bike lights are compact, reliable, powerful and inexpensive. Front lights usually attach to your handlebars, back lights fasten to your seatpost. Other mounting options are possible if that's a problem.

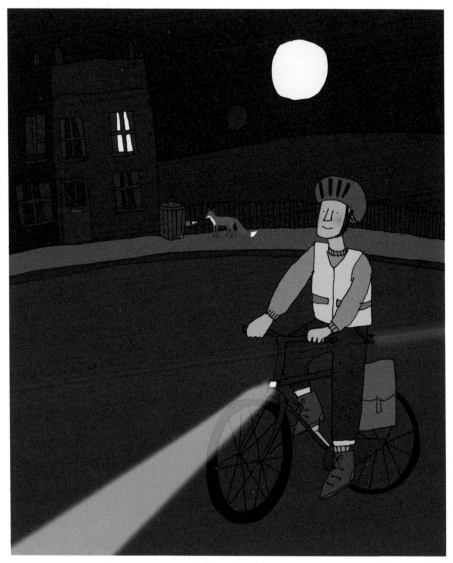

Clothing

The previous chapter looked at ways of making your bike more comfortable. What you wear can also make a significant difference. For short trips almost any sort of clothing will be fine but it's important to "bike-proof" it. Tie down or tuck in anything that might impede your control of the bike or get snagged in your wheels or chain. If you wear wide trousers the legs can be secured with Velcroed bands or cycle clips.

For longer journeys you might want to consider clothing tailored specifically for cycling. Such designs have many useful features. Seams will be positioned where they don't chafe your skin and cause soreness. Garments will be cut with cycling in mind: you change shape slightly when you lean forward to reach the handlebars so sleeves will be a little longer while jackets will be a tad shorter at the front and longer at the rear so that the small of your back is covered. Trousers or leggings will have an extra seam at the knee to allow for the bending and flexing that goes with pedalling. Pockets will be easy to reach on the move and may have tabs on the zips so that they can be opened and closed while wearing gloves. Cycling clothes tend to be made from fabrics that are soft and stretchy. They move with you, eliminating irritation and soreness, and they wick perspiration away keeping you cool and comfortable. There's gear galore to kit you out from top to toe. Let's start at the top:

Head

In the cycling world there is an ongoing discussion – to put it mildly – about the benefits of cycle helmets and whether people should be encouraged or even compelled to wear them. At present, helmets are optional in the UK. [19]

Advocates of helmets see them as a common-sense safety measure that can reduce head injuries and save lives. The sceptics argue that the amount of protection provided by a cycle helmet is routinely overstated. They point to countries like Denmark and the Netherlands where comparatively few people wear helmets, yet cycling is many times safer than in the UK. Good facilities, they say, not compulsion, is the way to go. Examine the arguments for and against by visiting www.cycle-smart.org (pro) and www.cyclehelmets.org (anti).

---

19   Since June 2014, children under the age of 14 on the Channel Island of Jersey (a British Crown dependency, not in the UK) must wear a cycle helmet.

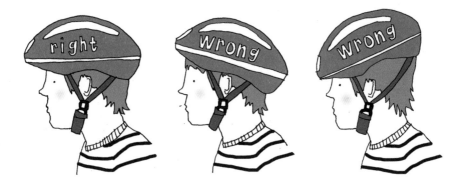

If you choose to wear a cycle helmet, do four things:

- **Buy a quality product.** Check that the helmet has a CE mark and that it meets at least one recognised standard, either BS EN 1078: 1997 (the European standard) or Snell B.95 (the American standard).
- **Wear it properly.** Buy a helmet that's the right size. Put the helmet on, hold it firmly and try turning your head. If your head moves while the helmet stays still, the helmet is too big or too loose. The straps should be fastened snugly. The helmet should sit squarely on your head, never worn slung back like a cowboy hat or pulled rakishly forwards.
- **Be consistent.** It's totally illogical to wear a helmet for certain trips but not for others, or to take it off when the weather's warm and have it swinging from your handlebars. If you decide to wear a helmet, wear it for all journeys, however brief. Make it part of your cycling routine.
- **Be realistic.** A helmet does not make you invulnerable: it's not armour plating. Helmets are designed to offer some protection if you fall off your bike and bump your head. (Incidentally, if that does happen, the helmet will need to be replaced. As it will if you drop it onto a hard surface from a height of more than one-and-a-half metres). Wearing a helmet will not make you a more competent cyclist. It will not improve your control skills, enhance your judgment, or enable you to influence how other road users treat you. Cycle training, however, can have an effect on all of these things – as we shall see in Chapter Six.

Eyes
Sunglasses will protect your eyes against glare and they also guard against the peril of flying insects. As well as dark designer shades bike shops sell protective specs with clear lenses for use on duller days.

Neck and ears

In a chilly wind, don't underestimate how cold and achy your ears can get. Covering them up from the start of your ride can make a big difference. Earmuffs and scarves are available in different weights and are perfect for keeping your neck and ears warm.

Upper body

You soon warm up when you're cycling so you need less clothing than you might imagine. That chunky cable-knit sweater might seem essential when you first emerge from the house but after a few miles I guarantee you'll be taking it off and wondering where to put it. The best way to control your body temperature is to wear several thin layers and then add or remove items to get the temperature balance right.

On cold days wear soft, porous layers close to your skin and wear something windproof and breathable as an outer "shell". The base layer provides insulation and the shell keeps the warmth in. You'll stay a lot more comfortable if your outer shell layer has a good degree of breathability. This is especially important for rainwear. If your perspiration vapour can't exit through the pores of the fabric it will condense and you'll quickly become hot and bothered, sticky and sore. Gore-Tex is the most famous breathable fabric but there are several other brands. If the high-tech approach doesn't appeal try waxed cotton or simply go for roomy outer garments with vents that aid airflow.

Hands

Even on bright spring mornings your hands can become chilled to the point of pain amazingly quickly. Gloves, of course, are the solution. They need to be thick enough to keep your hands warm, yet thin enough for you to flex your fingers, change gear, and brake properly. Gloves lined with materials such as Thinsulate do the job.

Gloves can also protect your hands against vibration. The ulnar nerve that runs from your hand up the length of your arm can become inflamed by vibration, especially if you hold your hand in a single position for long periods. So gloves, or fingerless mitts, with gel padding are a good idea whatever the weather.

Bottom

Some people seem able to hop onto a bike – any bike – and ride long distances in total comfort. Others find that even short rides leave them wincing, and walking like John Wayne after crossing the High Sierras. Take heart: saddle soreness can be prevented. Find a saddle that's right for you, set it to the correct height (see Chapter Four), wear shorts or leggings that are designed for cycling and that are padded in the appropriate places and you'll be fine.

Proper cycling shorts have a padded seat and are made from six or eight pieces (or panels) of stretchy, figure-hugging Lycra (also known as Spandex or elastane). Eight-panel shorts offer the best fit. Lycra cycle shorts are meant to be worn (yikes!) without underwear.

One drawback of figure-hugging Lycra is that it's very revealing. If you're not blessed with the contours of a ballerina you might prefer to be a little more discreet. Try wearing cycling undershorts in place of your normal underwear. These are tailored and padded in the same way as shorts, and are topped off with conventional shorts, trousers or a skirt.

Legs

Trousers designed for the bike have a padded seat and seams that are positioned so that they don't cause discomfort. All sorts of styles are available including formal office-wear, chinos and denim jeans. There are trousers in thermal materials for cold winters and lightweight fabrics for summer. Some have water repellent qualities. If the weather gets really stormy there are waterproof over-trousers. You'll find those in breathable GoreTex the most comfortable for long periods.

Stretchy tights are an alternative to trousers. They're light and very comfortable but tend to give men the look of a stick insect when worn off the bike. Again, there are thermal designs for chilly days. You can also choose tights with a bib, providing additional warmth to your torso.

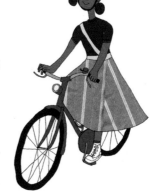

Skirts. Now, I'm not an authority on this subject but I have been advised that it's easy to cycle, even in a long flowing skirt, given a spot of practice and preparation. Here are some tips:
- A "ladies" bike, that's one with an open step-through frame (see Chapter Three), is best.
- A short skirt is easier to ride in than a longer one. If you do opt for a long skirt, a mesh skirt-guard over the back wheel will prevent it catching in the

spokes. A chain-guard stops it getting munched up by the chain.

- Skirts with a spot of Lycra in the weave, or with pleats, make pedalling easier. Tight fitting pencil shirts are the most difficult to ride in.
- Chose quality underwear. It may come under public scrutiny.
- Practise deportment: that's getting on and off the bike, moving off, and standing on the pedals when going uphill. These are critical moments so far as your dignity is concerned.

Feet

Any sort of shoe is fine for cycling so long as it allows you to keep your feet on the pedals and to slide them off again when you need to. If you're cycling in a skirt (see above) you may want to complete the outfit by wearing stilettos or platform soled shoes. I'm told that it's perfectly possible but I can't bring myself to recommend it. If you must have a heel, wedges are the more practical option. Better still, ride in flat shoes and carry your posh ones in a pannier. Change on arrival.

Fitting toe clips enables you to apply power on the upstroke (the pull) as well as the downstroke (the push) of the pedals, a technique the pros call "spinning." This makes for greater efficiency. If you use toe clips you'll need shoes that can slide out of the clip very quickly. Get someone to hold your bike upright and practise the technique before setting off for a ride.

Actually, toe clips are rather passé these days. They've been superseded by "clip-less" pedals. The mechanism is based on ski boot bindings. Special shoes and pedals are required. The shoes have a metal cleat in the sole that clips into a slot in the pedal. You're then attached to the bike, and rider and machine move as one. It's a great feeling, if a little scary at first. To release the clip, you twist your heel outwards and the cleat detaches. Again, practice is vital. All kinds of footwear are available with the built-in cleats for clipless cycling. There are canvas sneaker style shoes, clumpy boots for off-road riding, even sandals.

Just as your fingers are vulnerable to cold, your toes are too. Wear appropriate socks: thermal in winter, lightweight in summer. There are waterproof socks for rainy days or you can use gaiters or overshoes.

If you're riding at night, in traffic or in murky weather conditions bright, or better still, fluorescent clothing makes sense. I know people who cycle absolutely **everywhere** wearing fluorescent **everything.** The effect is eye-catching bordering on the terrifying.

48

A degree of fluorescence is just as effective and far more tasteful. Some jackets and tops intended for cycling have reflective strips cunningly incorporated into the design. Alternatively, you can add fluorescence by donning a reflective tabard or sash. These items can then be taken off and folded away when you reach your destination. Many local councils' road safety departments have high visibility items available at low cost.

Many mountain bikers sport a "skunk stripe" of muck up their backs as a kind of badge of honour. If you prefer to stay clean on your bike and to protect your outfit from road spray, make sure that your bike is fitted with mudguards. They are usually standard equipment on city bikes, tourers and hybrids. If they're not, it's quite easy to add them. Your local bike shop will do it for you. Choose mudguards that fasten to the frame with substantial metal stays rather than plastic clip-on guards which have a habit of shaking loose.

Ready... 6

If you're going for a ride you need a reliable bike that's set up properly and hopefully the advice in Chapter Three (remember the M-shaped bike check?) has got that side of things sorted. In this chapter we'll get **you** ready for the road.

Before you take up cycling or, indeed, embark on any programme of exercise it's wise to discuss your intentions with your GP. This is particularly important if you are overweight, unfit, if you haven't exercised for a while, if you have a particular medical condition, or if you suffer any persistent aches and pains. Your doctor may want to give you an examination to check your general state of health and may offer some additional lifestyle advice about matters such as diet, smoking and (sorry about this) alcohol consumption. Many medics these days are cyclists themselves so you're likely to find them very supportive.

If you're not used to exercise you may find that your first bike ride feels awkward and uncomfortable and you'll be surprised how inflexible your body feels. People who are already active – who walk, swim, play sport or go to exercise classes, for example – will fare better. But everyone is likely to benefit from a few preparatory exercises before getting on the bike. These are simple, gentle movements designed to wake up your metabolism and slowly get your body ready for an increased level of activity. There are two stages: a warm-up, and then a few stretches. Both, by the way, are beneficial if done at the end of a bike ride too, a practice known as "warming down." It will help your body return to normal and can prevent subsequent stiffness and twinges.

Warm up
Warm-up exercises prepare the muscles and joints for the work ahead and promote blood circulation. As the name suggests, they raise your body temperature a little, making the muscles more flexible and receptive to activity. Warming up should slightly increase your breathing and heart rate.

Here are five easy warm-up exercises. Try and do all of them. Ideally, work them into a short routine of five to 10 minutes. If you find it too strenuous, do less or allow yourself more time. Doing them to a lively piece of music gives everything a rhythm and makes it more enjoyable. Close the curtains if you're feeling self conscious!

Marching on the spot
Keep going for 3 minutes

Step smartly up and down lifting your knees almost to waist height. Pump your arms up and down in rhythm with your steps. Keep your elbows bent and your fists soft. Try marching forwards and then backwards a metre or so if you can.

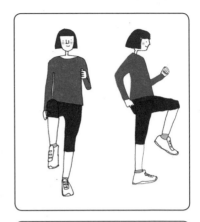

Heel digs
Aim for 60 heel digs in 60 seconds

Push one heel in front of you. Push it firmly against the floor with the toes pointing upward. Push your gently clenched fists forward with each heel dig. Keep a slight bend in the supporting leg.

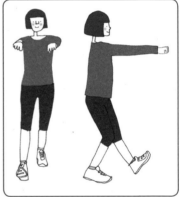

Knee lifts
Aim for 30 knee lifts in 30 seconds

Stand upright and raise alternate knees to touch the hand on the opposite side of your body (left knee to right hand, right hand to left knee, and so on). Keep your abdominal muscles tight and your back straight. Keep the supporting leg slightly bent.

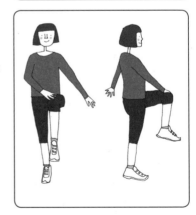

Shoulder rolls
2 sets of 10 repetitions

Do this one sitting down if you wish. Sit, or stand up, straight. Lift and roll your shoulders forwards and then backwards in a circular motion. Begin with little circles and progress to larger ones. Be gentle and take it slowly: don't force anything.

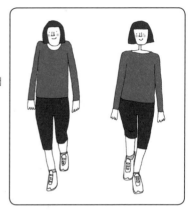

Knee bends
10 repetitions

Stand with your feet apart and your hands stretched out. Lower yourself no more than four inches or 10cm by bending your knees. Rise up and repeat.

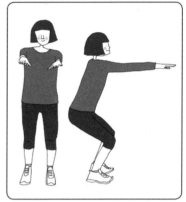

Stretches
After warming up, try some of these stretching exercises. They are designed to help increase the elasticity and strength of many of the muscles you use when cycling. Fitness instructors would advise you to do each stretch for 20 to 60 seconds and to perform each one two to four times. Choose three or four stretches from the 12 listed below and work them into a routine that lasts 10 to 15 minutes. Pick a different selection for another 15-minute session to do on another day. Gaining flexibility is a long-term process. Four 15-minute sessions over a week is better than an hour-long session once a week.

As with the warm-up exercises, if you find it too strenuous, do less or allow yourself more time.

Stretch slowly without bouncing or jerking. Don't try to force your body into position and don't worry about how far you can stretch: suppleness develops over time with regular stretching. Stretch to the point of feeling a slight tension or a pull on the muscle at the peak of the stretch. Never stretch to the point of pain: if it hurts, you're over-stretching. And don't forget to breathe – deeply and evenly throughout. Never hold your breath while you stretch.

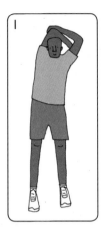 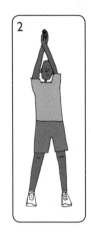 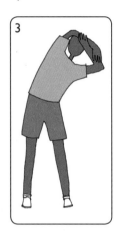 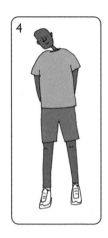

1 : Arms and tops of shoulders
Fold your arms behind your head. Grab one elbow and gently pull it. Refrain from bending at the waist and from jerking your elbow when you apply pressure to it. Swap arms and repeat.

2 : Arms, shoulders and outer chest
With your legs a shoulders'-width apart, reach out above your head and reverse your hands. Then stretch upwards and slightly backwards, keeping your feet flat on the floor.

3: Outer shoulders and chest
With legs a shoulders'-width apart, put your arms together as pictured, keeping your hands flat and relaxed. Bend sideways at the waist and hold for 10 seconds. Relax and repeat, bending the opposite way.

4: Neck
Sit or stand in a comfortable and upright position and stare straight ahead. Move your head slowly from side to side slowing stretching the muscles. Keep your

shoulders relaxed and steady and resist the temptation to jerk your head. Repeat 10 times.

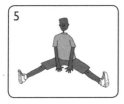 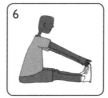 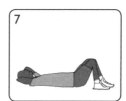 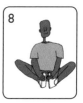

5 : Groin and inner thighs

Sit down with your knees locked and spread as far apart as possible. Relax and reach forward, slowly bending at the waist. Hold this for 10 seconds. Then slowly turn and face one foot and reach towards your ankle or lower leg. Hold this for a further 10 seconds, sit back and repeat, turning to the other leg.

6 : Hamstrings

Sit down with legs together and straight out in front of you. Reach forward with both hands and attempt to touch your toes. Don't force it. Remember you should be able to feel muscles stretching but it should not be painful.

7 : Lower back

Lie on your back with your knees raised, feet flat against the floor, should-width apart and hands clasped behind your head. Flatten your back against the floor by tensing your buttocks and abdominal muscles.

8 : Groin

Sitting, with the soles of your feet flat together grasp your toes. Gentle pull the toes whilst leaning forward and pushing your knees down with your elbows. Hold for 10 seconds, then relax.

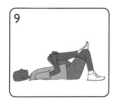 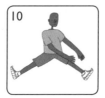 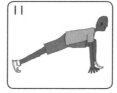 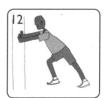

9 : Buttocks and hips

Lie down and keep one foot flat on the floor. Bring the other leg up and pull it toward the chest, grasping it below the knee with fingers clasped. Hold for 10 seconds, relax, then repeat with the other leg.

10 : Ankles
Sit with your legs spread in front of you. Rotate one ankle as far as it will go both ways. If you can reach, apply gentle pressure with the opposite hand. Repeat 10 times then swap ankles.

11 : Hips and thighs
Adopt a lunge position. Place your right foot flat in front of you and move it forward until the knee is above the ankle and the hind knee is touching the floor. Balance with your hands on the floor, keep both feet pointing straight ahead and move your hips forward. Swap sides.

12 : Calves
Stand close to the wall or some kind of vertical support, placing your hands a shoulders'-width apart and flat against it with elbows slightly bent. Place one leg in front of you and, with your hind hell flat, move your hips forward and hold. Swap legs and repeat.

As well as getting your body ready for cycling you also need to prepare mentally. Unless you're fortunate enough to have a network of traffic-free cycle trails on your doorstep you're likely to encounter traffic at some point during your rides. Many new cyclists find the prospect intimidating and returnees are often surprised by the degree to which motor traffic has grown over the years.

According to the Department for Transport there are now more than 34-million motor vehicles jostling for space on this small island of ours. Even so, traffic need not be a barrier to getting out on your bike. Busy roads can often be avoided. Even in the most congested cities there are usually quiet back streets and lightly trafficked roads that are fine for cycling. You can also exploit routes that aren't available to motorists: cycle tracks, canal towpaths and shortcuts through parks and other open spaces. Routes of this type don't just help you escape the town and find open country; they're often pleasant riding in their own right.

If getting out of town by bike really isn't an option, or if you want to explore more distant places, you might be able to jump-start your journey by using a car or public transport for the first leg. Folding bikes are ideal for this. A folder will go in the boot of a car or into a railway carriage with you. Folders can go by bus too, although few bus companies officially allow it and some drivers can be difficult. The trick is to bag it up (a bin liner will do) and pretend that the bike is just another piece of luggage.

Full sized bikes can also go by train although the various rail operators all have different rules as to how many bikes they take and whether you need to make an advance booking. Check out the rules at your local station's travel centre. There's also useful info on A to B magazine's website.

With a bit of ingenuity (removing the front wheel, for example) and a sheet to protect your upholstery it's often possible to get a full-sized bike inside a car. Or you can buy an external carrier rack. There are three main types: racks that clip around the lid of the boot or rear hatch and rest on the back of the car, roof racks, and racks that fit on the car's tow-bar or tow-ball. To be street-legal the racks and bikes need to be firmly attached with no protrusions that might strike a pedestrian or fellow road user. Your view of the road, including through your rear view mirror, should not be obscured. Ensure that the car's lights and rear number plate are clearly visible.

Even if you do have to mix with a little traffic on your bike ride it might not be as problematic as you first thought. You can cope if you have the skill and the confidence – and the key to acquiring both is Bikeability training.

Unlike Bikeability for children (which we looked at in Chapter Two) adult courses are usually run on a one-to-one basis. That's you and your instructor. Forget the old-fashioned Cycling Proficiency course that you might have gone through as a child. Adult Bikeability is dignified and discreet training for grown-ups. One of the benefits of the one-to-one format is that lessons are tailored to your particular needs and concerns, and you will never be pushed beyond your abilities. If you have a particular medical condition for example, your trainer will take that into account. If you're a nervous slow learner that's not a problem. Think of your Bikeability instructor as a sympathetic friend, a brain to pick, a source of sound advice and wise counsel.

For beginners there's off-road training to instil basic skills and to build confidence. This takes place in a quiet traffic-free area such as a park. Over time, if you wish, you can graduate to quiet roads and learn how to move off, maintain a straight line, pass parked cars, give hand signals, turn left and right and handle a variety of traffic conditions. Your instructor will show you how seemingly simple things, such as where your position yourself on the road, can have a substantial influence on the way other road users treat you.

Most towns now run adult Bikeability courses. They may be provided by the local council or by independent companies or charities. In London and many other areas there's an emerging market in cycle training and there are several providers to choose from. The Bikeability website enables you to search for your nearest provider. Lessons are often subsidised, or may even be free of charge.

Before their training many people are somewhat sceptical. Afterwards they're exuberant. The whole experience of riding in traffic suddenly feels so much easier. I know of at least one Bikeability provider that offers a money back guarantee. Course fees are refunded if trainees considered the training anything less than life changing. Even after several thousand bookings they have never had to give a refund.

Steady...

With your body, brain and bicycle roadworthy, it's time to plan a ride. If you're new to cycling or if you're not particularly fit you might want to begin with a few circuits round a local park (check that cycling is permitted), or round your neighbourhood on cycle paths and quiet roads. Your local council probably publishes a cycle map that will help you find these routes. Short rides of this type are good exercise and they might be the limit of your ambition – and that's absolutely fine. But as your ability and stamina improve – and they will the more you practise – you may want to venture further afield.

When planning a more ambitious bike ride, choose a route that is well within your capabilities. For beginners and people who are not particularly fit I recommend:

- Lightly-trafficked roads or traffic-free cycle trails or a mixture of the two.
- Flattish, or gently rolling terrain. Steep hills and rough tracks will slow you down and you may find them hard going.
- A manageable distance. This a bit of a moveable feast because everyone is different. How far you'll ride depends on your how fit you are, the nature of the terrain and the clemency of the weather. Fit, sporty types can easily average 15 miles per hour or more, so in a day they'll cover... well, you work it out. Ordinary mortals average less than 10 mph. If you take into account breaks for refreshments, adding or removing items of clothing, checking the map, picking blackberries, or admiring the view – all of which are to be heartily encouraged, by the way – then you may only cover five miles every hour. This is nothing to apologise for. Comfort, rather than speed or distance, should be your priority.

Most people prefer a circular to a linear ride because the scenery constantly changes, you cover more ground and you get a nice feeling of accomplishment at the end. Yet linear rides have a lot to commend them too, which is just as well because if you want a route that's completely traffic free, a railway path or similar linear trail is often the only option. It's seldom a second-rate experience though. Even though you cover the ground twice – there and back again – it rarely feels repetitious because you get to take in the view from different angles, and you'll spot things on the return journey that you missed on the way out. It's hard to get lost on a linear route and distances are always under your control. If you've had enough or you're starting to tire simply turn round and head back.

Here are some organisations that will help you find a great place to cycle (contact details are in the back of the book):

Local councils. Many areas have a flagship "cycleway" designed for leisure cycling. Try a Google search for the word "cycleway" and you'll see some examples (the Wiltshire Cycleway, the Lancashire Cycleway, etc). Usually on quiet roads and traffic-free tracks, they take you round the county through some of its finest scenery. The entire circuit will probably be too much to do in a single day but it's often possible to devise a ride that takes in sections of the route. When you hit the road you'll find helpful signposts to keep you on track. To help you plan there are usually free maps available from libraries, tourist information offices, or from the cycling pages of the council's website. Take a look at the "Cycle A-way" section of the CTC website too. It lists all the published cycle routes in the British Isles and tells you how to get hold of the relevant maps.

Sustrans (short for sustainable transport) is the charity behind the UK's 14,000-mile National Cycle Network (NCN). The organisation claims that half the UK population lives within one mile of its routes. The NCN is designed to be family friendly and easy to ride. Almost a third of the network is traffic free, using railway paths, riversides or forest trails. The rest is on roads but hundreds of cycle lanes, signal-controlled crossings and bridges have been built so that you rarely have to mix with heavy traffic. Many of the routes have alluring names such as the Cuckoo Trail, the Centurion Way and the Sea to Sea (or C2C for short) and they're all numbered and signposted. The Sustrans website lets you search for routes by postcode, route number, terrain (you can look for forests, lakes or coastal routes) or by ease of use (you can specify "easy ride" or "traffic free"). Plan a route on your computer and then print a map. Alternatively, there's a vast range of maps, leaflets and guidebooks available from the Sustrans on-line shop.

The Canal & River Trust, the successor to British Waterways, cares for most of the country's canals and many of its rivers. Alongside each waterway, there's usually a path, and the majority are open to cyclists. The quality is variable. Some are narrow, muddy and rutted; others have a smoother surface and enough space for walkers, cyclists and anglers to co-exist peacefully. Apart from the odd flight of locks, there are no real hills to worry about. Such paths are easy to follow: if there's water to one side of you, you're on track. Canals tend to pass through towns and villages at regular intervals and are dotted with pleasant waterside pubs, so there are usually lots of refreshment opportunities.

According to the Canal & River Trust, 21-million cycle trips are made on the nation's waterside routes every year, proof that the mixture of attractive scenery, boats, wildlife and industrial history has a powerful appeal.

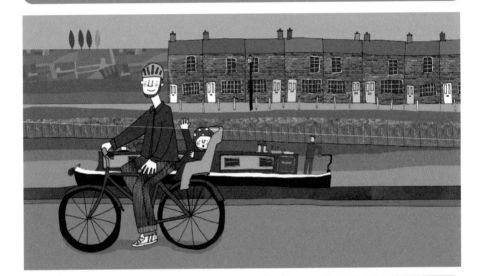

Forests. Forestry Commission (England), Forestry Commission (Scotland), Natural Resources Wales, and the Northern Ireland Forest Service collectively look after many thousands of hectares of woodland, and most of their forest tracks are open to cyclists. Surfaces can be rough at times and although the trails are generally traffic free you need to keep an eye out for the occasional logging truck or Land Rover. Otherwise, expect stunning scenery, majestic trees, fresh air, squirrels, deer, butterflies, birdsong and wildflowers. If you don't want to plan your own route, many forests have waymarked trails to meet just about everyone's needs: short routes for beginners and family groups, longer rides for more experienced cyclists, through to rollercoaster courses for hardcore mountain bikers. The New Forest, the Forest of Dean, Thetford Forest, Coed Y Brenin, Glentress Forest and many others have a bike hire centre, complete with café, toilets, and shop.

The National Trust cares for miles of coastline, country estates, forests and moorland as well as mansions, castles and other properties throughout England, Wales and Northern Ireland. There's a separate National Trust for Scotland. Cycling is encouraged and many properties have waymarked trails. Some are specifically designed with children in mind. One-in-six National Trust properties, from historic houses to glorious gardens, offers visitors who arrive without a car a discount on their entry fee or a voucher that you can spend in one of their excellent tea-rooms.

Ordnance Survey or OS for short is a cartographer rather than a landowner - and a national treasure. The OS has mapped the whole of the UK in fantastic detail. You can buy their maps from most bookshops and outdoor stores, or from the OS website and other on-line retailers. Alternatively, borrow them free of charge from most public libraries. The Landranger series of maps (pink cover) has a scale of 1:50,000 (two centimetres to the kilometre), while the Explorer series (orange cover) has a more comprehensive 1:25,000 scale (four centimetres to the kilometre). The quiet lanes sought after by cyclists are the C-class roads, shown as yellow lines. It takes time to get really good at map reading but it's a rewarding skill to develop. With practice you become adept at spotting places of interest (ancient burial mound anyone?) and getting a feel for the rise and fall of the terrain and the character of the landscape.

As well as Ordnance Survey publications there are numerous other maps and guides available that will help you find easy bike rides in picturesque places. You can also get ideas from cycling websites, bike magazines and Sunday newspapers.

Electronic mapping is gaining in popularity. Lots of cars have GPS (Global Positioning System) or SatNav systems and the same technology can be utilised by cyclists. GPS units from the likes of Garmin or Memory-Map enable you to plan a route on your computer and then transfer the data to the unit. Clip it to your handlebars and off you go. The device will guide you on your way and you'll always know exactly where you are – that means less time poring over a paper map and more time enjoying the journey.

GPS units are getting cheaper but even entry level models cost over £100. An alternative and cheaper way of getting route info electronically is to use a smartphone with a handlebar mounting. There are various on-line journey planners that are free to use, or you can download cycle-specific apps that will find you a route that best meets your particular needs. For example, you can stipulate the most direct, the quietest or the least hilly route, or search for bike shops and other points of interest on the way.

When setting off for your ride it's important to dress for the weather. We looked at some clothing options in Chapter Five. This being Britain, the weather can change quite dramatically in the blinking of an eye so, as well as a quick look outside, it's wise to check the Met Office forecast for the day. If you decide it's time to unleash your summer outfit pack a tube of sunscreen too and make regular use of it. When you're cycling there's a constant flow of cool air over your body and you may be unaware of the fact that you're getting sunburnt. All your exposed bits, and even bits covered by light clothing, are vulnerable.

Dehydration can sneak up on you in a similar way to sunburn. When you cycle the combination of raised metabolism and airflow means you can dry out rapidly, often without realising. You might not even feel thirsty. The consequences of dehydration can be quite serious, but fortunately the problem can be prevented by – you've got it! – drinking water. Little and often is the way to go. Fit a bottle cage to your bike so you can keep a supply to hand. Tap water is fine, as is bottled water (the body prefers still to fizzy) or fruit squash. A break at a good tea shop or café is one of the delights of a bike ride, but don't rely solely on tea and coffee for refreshment; they're fine in moderation but they can speed up the dehydration process. Alcohol does too – and it will impair your ability to control the bike. Save that celebratory glass for the evening.

I mentioned tea shops and cafés. These, along with pubs, village shops, bakeries, farmers' markets and the occasional church fete are fantastic opportunities to rest and refuel, and to inject a little money into the local economy. A word or two of caution though; even if your map promises a pub or a shop don't rely on it actually being there. Businesses disappear or have strange opening hours, kitchen staff go on holiday or shops run out of stock. Instead of that delicious lunch you promised yourself in a half-timbered gastro-pub, you might end up sitting in a draughty bus shelter with a bag of Cheesy Wotsits from a petrol station.

On the other hand, if your chosen route is strewn with inviting eateries, there's always the temptation to overindulge. Exercise and fresh air are famous for stimulating the appetite, but take in too many cream teas or heavy lunches and any hopes you had of losing weight will be dashed. On top of that, a blowout followed by a bike ride can lead to indigestion and a bloated, sluggish feeling that spoils the rest of the day. The trick is to keep your appetite under control: not too full, not too hungry. Begin the day with a decent breakfast and when you set off on your ride, make sure you've got some food with you. Flapjacks, cereal bars and bananas are many a cyclist's snack of choice. Dried fruit, seeds and nuts are also good. They don't take up much room and they won't come to harm at the bottom of your bag. These light nibbles will help you maintain your energy levels and keep hunger pangs at bay.

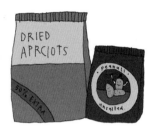

You'll benefit from snacks – and, indeed, main meals – that are light on fat, sugar, salt and protein and stronger on carbohydrate, especially the unrefined sorts. Starchy foods such as jacket potatoes, brown rice, wholemeal bread and pasta release their energy gradually, meaning that you feel fuller for longer and less inclined to over-eat. Mention brown rice to some people and they tend to get a bit depressed but it's really just a matter of balance: enjoy a few treats by all means but make them part of a diet that's rich in fruit, veg, fibre and carbs as well.

A well maintained bike is a superbly reliable machine and mechanical problems are unlikely out on your ride. But it's advisable to prepare for the worst. Even if you're not sure how to use them, carry a pump, a spare innertube and a multi-tool with you. Multi-tools are nifty, all-purpose gadgets for tightening up any nuts or bolts that may come loose and to effect a few quick repairs. [20] A typical example contains the following implements:

- Allen keys (eight different sizes)
- Spanners (three different sizes)
- A special spanner for removing pedals
- Flat and cross-head screwdrivers
- A chain-removing tool
- A couple of tyre levers
- A spoke adjustment key

You might be unlucky and get a puncture. We talk about a punctured tyre but it's actually the innertube inside the tyre which holds the air and gives you a smooth ride, and if it's pricked the tube/tyre combo goes flat. Never ride with a flat tyre: it

---

20   A multi-tool also has all you'll need to assemble flat-packed furniture!

will damage the wheel. In town punctures are invariably caused by shards of broken glass, out in the countryside the culprit is more likely to be a thorn. If your tyre goes flat you have various options.

Try pumping up the tyre.
- How easy? Easy.
- Requirements? Pump.
- Chances of success? 50/50 Although it's still leaking, the tube may hold enough air to let you cycle a few more miles, and, possibly with repeated pumpings, enable you to complete the ride or reach assistance.

Change the tube.
- How easy? Moderate.
- Requirements? Tyre levers. Spare inner-tube. Pump. Multi-tool to undo the wheelnuts (if your bike doesn't have quick-release fastenings).
- Chances of success? 100% However, you'll need to know how to remove the wheel and you'll need the skill and the strength in your fingers to lever off the tyre and extract the punctured tube. Feel about inside the tyre and find the thorn or piece of glass that caused the puncture. Remove it. Fit the spare tube, refit the tyre, put the wheel back on and inflate. Take the damaged tube home for repair.

Repair the puncture.
- How easy? Moderate to quite tricky.
- Requirements? Puncture repair kit. Pump. Multi-tool.
- Chances of success? 100% so long as the tyre has only been pricked or received a tiny cut. A large gash is a lost cause. Whip off the wheel, remove the tyre, pull out the inner tube, find the puncture, remove that pesky thorn or shard, and apply a patch. Check the inside of the tyre for any other debris that might damage the tube. Put everything back together again and pump it up. There are books that will teach you how to mend a puncture or you can find step-by-step instructions, for free, on the internet. You may also find that local cycling groups run courses, or you may have a friend, relative or colleague who could teach you. Give it a go. Master puncture repair and you've learnt a valuable skill.

Call for assistance.
- How easy? Simple.
- Requirements? Membership of roadside recovery organisation. Phone. Phone signal.

- Chances of success? 100% (although you may have to wait for a while). The Environmental Transport Association (ETA) sees itself as the Green equivalent of the AA or the RAC. Like those organisations it provides services for motorists but it also offers a roadside recovery service for cyclists. If your bike develops a problem – even something as simple as a puncture – and you're unable to complete your journey an ETA patrol will take you and your bike to a nearby railway station, cycle repair shop, hotel or – if feasible – back home.

Stop a cyclist.

- How easy? Easy. As long as you can find one.
- Requirements? Confidence. A winning smile.
- Chances of success? High. In this hard-edged uncaring age, when neighbours barely know each other and strangers are viewed with suspicion, there's still a surprising degree of camaraderie out on the open road. Other cyclists are likely to be sympathetic to the plight of a fellow traveller and be happy to help out. Cycle tourists or seasoned commuters (look for the fluorescent clothing, the classy bike, the bulging panniers) will probably have a full set of tools and be willing to help you with the repair or even do it for you.

We're almost ready for that bike ride. Here's a handy checklist to make sure you're properly prepared:

Bike ride checklist

In advance
☐ Bike checked and declared roadworthy
☐ Weather forecast checked
☐ Route planned

Packed
☐ Suitable clothes (wet weather gear if appropriate)
☐ Sunscreen and sunglasses if necessary
☐ Simple first aid kit
☐ Cash and credit cards
☐ Phone
☐ Toolkit
☐ Pump, spare inner tube and multi-tool.
  Any other tools and spares that you know how to use.

☐ Maps or guidebook
    (even if you're following a signposted route, take a map. Signs sometimes go missing.)
☐ Food
☐ Water
☐ Bike lock (and the key!)
☐ Lights if there's a chance that you'll be out after dark

That might seem a vast amount of stuff but it actually makes for quite a compact bundle. Even so, if you're riding all day it's a pain to put it on your back in a rucksack. A set of panniers or some other luggage system that attaches to the bike (see Chapter Four) is the easiest way to carry it all.

Go!

And we're away! You're feeling a slight sense of trepidation as you set off, perhaps? The bike seems cumbersome and your arms and legs don't quite know what to do yet. This is entirely understandable. But if you can make it to the end of the road without falling off in front of the neighbours you'll begin to relax and to settle in to the rhythm of pedalling. In no time at all your cares vanish. Your focus is on the road ahead and your senses are busy taking in the scenery that's unfolding around you.

As you ride along there are a few things you can do to optimise your comfort.

Check that your saddle is at exactly the right height. We looked at setting the bike up properly in Chapter Four so everything should be broadly correct, but fine tuning is best done out on the road. If your saddle is too low your knees twist outwards which is uncomfortable and potentially damaging. Too high and you're stretching your knee joints, which is equally bad. Find a straight, level stretch of road and cycle along. If you think you need to raise the saddle, stop, flip the quick release fastening or undo the seatpost bolt with your multi-tool and alter the height of the saddle by a few millimetres. Retighten the fastening and ride on for a few minutes. Make repeated adjustments as required.

Teach yourself to ride lightly. If you see a rough bit of road ahead, freewheel. Rise up out of the saddle, lean forward a little and relax your arms and legs slightly. Keep hold of the handlebars, but loosely, not in a death grip. The bike will clatter over the bumps but all the shock and vibration will be dispersed. The alternative, keeping your bottom stuck to the saddle, your neck and arms straight and your hands clamped tightly round the handlebars, means you feel every bump. The bike seems to be fighting you and it's an effort to retain control.

It can take time to develop the technique of riding light. If you're new to cycling you may not have sufficient strength in your leg muscles at first, but persevere. Get it right and you'll be able to cycle longer and further and you'll feel less tired at the end of the ride.

A quiet, level stretch of road is also a good place to practise your pedalling technique. Again, a light touch is required. Drivers are taught to work their way through the gears and get the car into top gear as soon as possible so that the engine isn't revving away and wasting fuel. You don't do this on a bike. Even though a high gear and a slow, steady pedalling cadence feel intuitive at first, it becomes tiring quite quickly. The human body likes lots of light, repetitive movements rather than fewer, more forceful ones. So choose a slightly lower gear. You'll push the pedals more rapidly but it will take less effort and it won't strain your knees. Once you've found a pedalling cadence that suits you, try to maintain it by using the gears, shifting up or down as the terrain changes.

You may have gears galore but there will still be hills that are too steep to ride up. You may have had Bikeability training (see Chapter Six) but you will still encounter busy junctions or stretches of road that you find unnerving. Well, it's fine to get off the bike and push. Cycling should be stress-free and (I've said this already) it shouldn't hurt. The macho mantra "no pain, no gain" is a silly falsehood. Don't force yourself beyond your abilities.

What if things go wrong? If the bike develops an insoluble problem, if the weather turns vile, or if you feel unwell, cut the ride short. The route will still be there to have a go at on another day; your well-being takes priority. It's no disgrace to turn tail and head home. Take a taxi if necessary. It's a little-known fact that most UK taxis will take bicycles, usually for a small additional charge. The classic black cab or a people carrier are your best bet. There are numerous smartphone apps that will find you a taxi anywhere in the world at any time of day. When booking the taxi make it clear that it's for you and a bicycle. Drivers may refuse to take your bike if it's crusted with mud or dripping oil, so try to spruce it up a bit while you're waiting for the cab to arrive.

A contingency plan is always a wise idea, but in truth you probably won't need it. I'm sure your ride will go splendidly. Savour the weather, the sights, sounds and smells. Explore, take detours, stop to look at things. If you need directions or your water bottle refilling, ask a local. Communities often regard cars as a nuisance and their occupants as noisy intruders, cyclists though are generally well received. Many a chance encounter on a bike ride has turned into a great conversation or even a lasting friendship.

That's it from me for this chapter. The rest is all about you. It's your adventure!

"...exercise and many drug interventions are often potentially similar in terms of their mortality benefits in the secondary prevention of coronary heart disease, rehabilitation after stroke, treatment of heart failure, and prevention of diabetes."

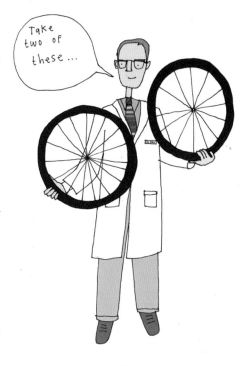

The extract above is taken from a study reported in the British Medical Journal.[21] It found that exercise can be as good as – or sometimes better than – drug treatment for people with conditions such as stroke or heart disease. And, unlike drugs, the researchers could find no significant side effects. The study looked at hundreds of trials involving nearly 340,000 patients to assess the merits of exercise and drugs in preventing death. The results were surprising. Physical activity rivalled some heart drugs and outperformed stroke medicine. The researchers concluded by suggesting that exercise should be added to prescriptions. It would be a win-win situation. Patients would gain a sense of empowerment and be able to take control of their treatment, while the hard-pressed NHS would save a fortune on its drugs bill.

The idea of cycling on prescription or on referral from a GP is not as fanciful as it might sound. Exercise on prescription initiatives are flourishing in many parts of the country. Some focus mainly on indoor activities such as dance, yoga and gym-based exercise. Others embrace the great outdoors as well and offer guided walks and a variety of bike-based activities.

---

21   British Medical Journal. 2013. Comparative effectiveness of exercise and drug interventions on mortality outcomes: metaepidemiological study. BMJ 2013; 347; f5577

In Croydon and Reading, for example, people with a medical condition, or who are overweight or just unfit can join weekly cycling for health sessions. They may get a referral from their GP or they can simply sign themselves up. People of all abilities are welcome, including complete beginners. The sessions are held in a safe, traffic-free space (the arena in Croydon, the velodrome in Reading) and a range of pedal-powered vehicles of various types – bikes, trikes, and recumbent cycles – are available to try out. The atmosphere is relaxed and informal: you grab a bike and have a go. Do as much as you want, at a pace you find comfortable. Friendly cycling advisers are on hand to provide support tailored to your individual needs. This can include Bikeability training, so that as your fitness and confidence grow you can improve your cycling skills and prepare for longer trips: a local charity ride perhaps, or the journey to work. The sessions also have a strong social aspect. You get to meet people in a similar situation to your own, who understand the problems and the issues you are dealing with. Hearing about their experiences can be a valuable aid to your own recovery.

Cycling Projects, based in the north-west of England, is an organisation with many years' experience of working with people who are recovering from, or who need to manage, a medical condition. They run rides for cardiac rehabilitation and weight management groups, and for people who simply want to keep fit and stay active while enjoying the freedom and fresh air of the outdoors. Many participants are referred to the rides by a GP or health specialist.

Novice cyclists are offered training to help develop their skills and confidence. There are also bike maintenance courses to teach people how to cope with a puncture and enable them to keep their bikes roadworthy. The rides take place on easy terrain on the growing network of traffic-free trails that criss-cross the north-west. Rides range from thirty minutes to an hour or more. Many hundreds of people have taken part and the results are impressive. Feedback from participants has been extremely positive with many people reporting that without the programme they would not have been able to take up cycling. As well as valuing the opportunity for regular exercise, participants tend to highlight the positive social components of the schemes, allowing them to swap stories and learn from other people in similar situations.

In Stockport, a number of cyclists with cardiac issues enjoyed the rides so much that they decided to set up their own group so that they could ride more frequently and maintain the friendships and mutual support that they felt to be so important to their rehabilitation. Thus, the Second Chance Cycling Club was born – an informal group open to anyone who has had heart problems and who wants to continue cycling. Membership is growing steadily.

In Bristol, the charity Life Cycle UK[22] runs three schemes with a health improvement dimension. Their **Silver Cyclists** programme of rides is aimed at over 55's who want to experience, or rediscover, the pleasures of cycling. The rides are moderately paced and use quiet roads and cycle tracks with strategic tea stops and café breaks factored in. They're led by trained ride leaders and supported by volunteers who are all experienced cyclists. People without bikes can borrow one; there's even the opportunity to try out an electric bike. Bikeability training is available, and there's the option of joining a class to learn basic cycle maintenance.

Life Cycle's **Bike Minded** initiative is a programme of group rides for people experiencing mental and emotional health issues such as anxiety, depression, sleep disorders, or addiction recovery. Mental health problems still carry a degree of stigma that makes it harder for those affected to hold down a job or enjoy an active social life. They may be reluctant to seek help, which makes recovery slower and more difficult. If they become housebound their physical health may decline. The Bike Minded rides are an opportunity to break this vicious circle and enjoy gentle exercise and a change of scene. People may self-refer to the project or be referred by mental health organisations, support workers and other agencies. The experience of riding with others in a calm, non-judgmental atmosphere brings results. One participant commented, "On a ride, I feel so 'normal' just chatting to people, without feeling like a mental health patient." Another said, "I have no doubt that the project has helped me return to work after over a year off – and remain in work." In a follow-up survey 67% of participants reported that they had made fewer trips to their GP as a result of their bike rides.

Many disabled people have very few opportunities to take exercise, and may experience weight gain, muscle wastage and poor circulation due to prolonged wheelchair use or a sedentary lifestyle. Yet even profound disability is no barrier to cycling. There are now scores of initiatives dedicated to helping people with disabilities or special needs to experience the freedom and exhilaration that comes with a bike ride. The rides are also opportunities for able-bodied people to ride with a disabled friend or family member.

---

22   Another fine cycling organisation that's been helping people take up cycling since 1996. I'm proud to have been its first Director.

I'll name just two such initiatives here. I'm deeply impressed with Cycling Projects' network of **Wheels for All** centres. They have a multitude of specially adapted bicycles, tricycles, hand-cranked cycles, wheelchair tandems and other vehicles designed for use by people with mobility issues. Experienced ride leaders and trainers are on hand to offer advice and to help participants get the most from every ride. There are now more than 50 Wheels for All centres across England and Wales.

Life Cycle's **Two's Company** project also deserves a mention; not least because I helped set it up! Thanks to a small fleet of tandems and an enthusiastic team of volunteer front-riders, blind and sight-impaired people in the Bristol area can experience a cycle ride and, as the name suggests, enjoy the company of others. Life Cycle runs at least 25 rides a year using local traffic-free routes like the famous Bristol and Bath railway path, as well as going further afield for an annual ride and barbecue in the Forest of Dean and a weekend of cycling and camping on the Tarka Tail in Devon. The youngest participant to date was just four years old, the oldest 76.

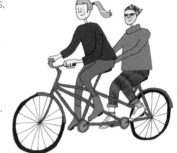

If you have a medical condition and you think cycling might be beneficial, make an appointment at your local surgery and discuss the idea with your GP, practice nurse or other healthcare professional. Don't just abandon your medication and reach for your cycle clips. If your doctor has prescribed a particular course of treatment they always have a good reason for doing so. But do ask whether cycling might improve your condition and, if so, whether you can be referred to a local scheme.

You might find that your doctor says yes to cycling, but doesn't know what's available in the way of help and support. That doesn't necessarily mean that nothing is happening in your area. A lot of cycling initiatives have a low profile and every area does its own thing. Whereas Bikeability is the national brand for cycle training, there's no similar brand name for cycling on prescription. Projects go under a variety of names and imaginative acronyms; I've discovered HEAL (Health, Exercise, Activity, Lifestyle), BITS (Back In the Saddle), HOW (Health On Wheels), and many more. Projects often rely on small amounts of short-term grant funding, so they tend to wax and wane. The ones mentioned above were all going strong at the time of writing (2015), but may not be around for ever.

As well as a strong, high profile brand, what's needed is a national, up-to-date, easy-to-use directory of cycling on prescription schemes. Until such a thing appears you'll need to do a bit of digging to find out what's available in your area. Try searching the internet for "cycling on prescription," "cycling on referral," "exercise on prescription," or "exercise on referral" followed by the name of your town. Try phoning the main switchboard of your local council and ask to speak to the person responsible for health improvement or health promotion. Or ask for the officer in the council's highways department who's responsible for cycling.

The UK has three national cycling organisations: CTC, Sustrans and British Cycling, and they may be able to help you. Sustrans for example has a network of "active travel champions" – volunteers who help people become more active by walking or cycling for some of their everyday journeys. Champions give advice and organise activities in their local community, workplace, university or school. CTC runs a Cycle Champions Programme with similar aims and has "cycling development officers" based regionally throughout the UK. The British Cycling website enables you to find bike-related events including rides for people with health-related needs. Use the website's search function. You'll find contact details for all these organisations at the back of the book.

Yes, it takes detective work to find a cycling for health scheme, but it's worth persisting. As you've probably noticed in the examples above, the schemes share certain ingredients. They're led by people who understand cycling and its health benefits and who appreciate the issues that newcomers face. They provide advice and support tailored to each individual's unique needs. Bikes and training are available. There are practice sessions in a safe, protected environment such as parks and green spaces. Then, if people are ready to venture further afield, there's a programme of rides that includes plenty of easy trips, over short distances, to attractive places. As well as being about bikes and cycling, the rides are about making friends, sharing experiences and providing mutual support. Mix in a generous dose of fun and this is powerful medicine.

I'm convinced that we're merely at the beginning and that cycling on prescription has vast potential. In time, even our slow-moving policy makers will have a eureka moment and wake up to the possibilities of cycling, both as preventative medicine, keeping us active and healthy from childhood into old age, and as a way of combating and managing a wide range of medical conditions. One day GP practices will double as cycling hubs with routes radiating outwards like a starburst. Experts will be on hand to offer guidance, bikes will be available to borrow, and there will be regular confidence boosting courses, guided rides and maintenance classes. Mark my words, this is the medicine of the future.

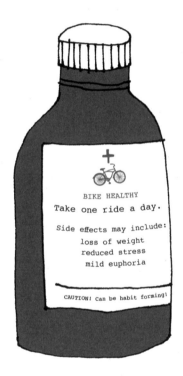

For cycling to work its magic, it needs to be done frequently. Two-and-half hours a week is the minimum dose.[23] More if you can. Even then, it won't deliver an immediate transformation. It will take time – several months maybe – before you'll feel genuinely fitter and can see a difference in the mirror. You need a degree of determination to maintain this level of activity and to resist the temptation to quit. A heavy cold, a series of rainy days, a couple of punctures, an encounter with a bad-mannered motorist... all sorts of things can scupper your initial enthusiasm and before you know it the bike gets consigned to the shed. The tyres go soft, the cobwebs bloom – and the pounds start to creep back on.

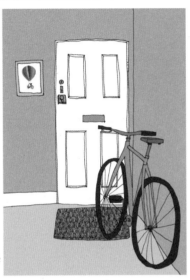

This chapter looks at some ways to increase your motivation, to ensure that you stay in the saddle and enjoy the benefits. The first is to make cycling into a habit, a part of your routine, and central to this is to keep your bike where it's easy to reach. If your nearest and dearest is amenable, consider storing your bike in the hallway, right by the front door where it's impossible to miss. The garage is a good second best – as long as the bike can be reached easily. If space is at a premium, you might want to invest in a cycle locker for the front garden. These are very secure cupboard-like storage units that take up to two bikes plus accessories.

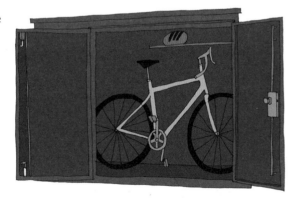

---

23   Just a reminder that this can be done as a series of short rides over the week. Re-read Chapter One for more information.

75

Embed cycling into your day. If you live within a reasonable distance from your workplace try commuting by bike. Not only will your health improve, you'll also save money on fares or fuel, and you'll probably have an easier, more reliable journey. Whereas the leisure cyclist (see Chapter Eight) has time to spare and relishes spontaneity, the commuter needs to more businesslike. Use some of the journey planning tools discussed in Chapter Ten to find potential routes and take time at the weekend or on an evening to ride them from home to work and then back again. Decide which route is likely to be the easiest and make a note of how long the journey takes. On Monday morning, when you ride it for real, allocate that amount of time plus about 30 percent to allow for busier conditions and unexpected delays.

Check out your workplace too. There has been a boom in cycle commuting over recent years and many employers have invested in bike parking, showers, lockers and other facilities to make cyclists welcome. If your employer isn't up to snuff see if they can be persuaded. There may be advice and grant aid available from your local council.

You can also use your bike for domestic errands such as shopping. Instead of driving to an edge-of-town retail park for a weekly supermarket-shop, pick up your groceries in smaller quantities on a more frequent basis. On a bike it's quick and easy to use local shops and markets as well as the bigger stores. You can normally park right outside your emporium of choice and be in and out in just a couple of minutes. You can access greater variety and get fresher food. Like commuting, a bike-based shopping trip quickly becomes a part of your routine, something to look forward to each time.

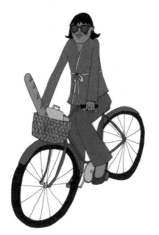

Strengthen your motivation by setting yourself a goal. It might be to increase your fitness, or to address a specific condition such as your weight or blood pressure or cholesterol level, or it might simply be to stay healthy. It might be to save money, to clock up so many miles, to see certain sights or to ride particular routes. Your goal should stretch you a bit but it must be something achievable. Choose goals based on interests and desires that are genuinely yours, don't just follow the crowd. Be realistic. Cycling can work wonders but it's unlikely to turn a 60-year-old into an Olympian or make you look 20 years younger. A brutal truth, I know, but there it is.

Break down your goal into a series of stages. This will make it feel less daunting and more achievable. Identify potential obstacles and think about how you'll get over them. Create a to-do list. Chapters Three to Eight of this book, which are all about preparation and planning, should help.

Be flexible. Life seldom goes exactly as planned so you should expect a few difficulties along the way. Revise your plans accordingly. It may take longer to reach your goal than you initially intended, but press on and you'll get there. Review your progress from time to time. All those items you've crossed off your to-do list are accomplishments. Well done you! A small reward is in order. Celebrate and then face up to the next challenge.

Goals are often easier to reach if they're underpinned with a numerical value. For many years time and distance were the only metrics in town. Now, we're inundated with gadgets that can record just about everything. There's tech that fastens to your bike or your body that will calculate calories consumed, heart-rate, blood pressure, pedalling cadence, speed (current, maximum and average), elevation, barometric pressure, as well as distance (total distance, trip distance) and time taken. Then, as we saw in Chapter Seven, there are GPS units and smartphone apps that will record your route in meticulous detail. There is, of course, such a thing as too much information, so be selective. Gather data that really means something, which you find genuinely interesting and that helps you understand your progress.

Record your achievements. The information gathered by your cycling gizmo or phone can usually be uploaded to a computer and expressed as graphs, charts, maps and spreadsheets. This is all useful stuff, but it's important to flesh out numerical data with thoughts and feelings. Call it what you will, a diary, a journal or log, do it on paper or electronically, but try to express in words what it is you're striving toward. On page one write down your goal and the steps required to reach it. Then record your rides, the highs and the lows, the lessons learned, the ideas that occurred to you along the way, the obstacles you've overcome, and the challenges you've still to address. Remind yourself of the value of what you're doing. Writing things down like this helps to make something abstract like "good health" feel real and it commits you to a course of action. It's like signing a contract with yourself.

Share your goal with others. Tell friends, family or work colleagues about your cycling

Psych for the bike! Try these motivational techniques.

Identify your goal.
It should personal to you, something you really care about. It should challenge you but be achievable.

Break it down.
Reduce your goal to a series of small steps.

Write it down.
Record your goal. Think about it, visualise it, imagine what reaching it will feel like. Write a to-do list.

Measure progress.
Use numbers, words and photographs. Keep a diary or blog, use social media or one of the many apps that let you record and monitor your cycling activity.

Involve others.
Share your goal with family and friends. Go cycling with others. Join a cycling club or your local cycling campaign.

Be flexible.
The best laid plans can go awry. Expect a few setbacks. Learn from your mistakes. Revise your plans as required.

Reward progress.
Congratulate yourself as you tick things off your to-do list. Treat yourself. A book or a film perhaps, or a massage, an item of clothing or a new piece of cycling kit.

Keep going!

goals. Articulating a goal out loud (or blogging it, or posting it on social media) will reaffirm your commitment and strengthen your resolve. It's a lot harder to back out of something that you've shared with other people. You know that they're going to ask how your cycling is going and that will help to keep you motivated.

Better still, go cycling with other people. This might mean simply getting together with a few friends on an informal basis, or joining a club or cycling campaign group. The UK's cycling clubs are thriving. There are elite clubs for high performance riders and, at the other end of the spectrum, laid-back groups that specialise in social rides over short distances. There are women-only groups and groups for middle-aged and older riders. More than 1,700 cycling clubs are affiliated to British Cycling and their website has a useful search function. Before joining a club ride, it's wise to contact the organiser and find out whether the distances they cover and the pace they go at are within your capabilities. Newcomers are usually welcome to join a ride, free of charge, to see whether they like it.

There are many good reasons for joining a cycling club or going on a group ride. There's the sense of camaraderie and there are opportunities to pick up tips and nuggets of information. If you have a cycling-related question there's likely to be someone in the group who knows the answer. You'll get to ride routes that are new to you and you can relax, knowing that the ride leader has (almost always) prepared carefully and knows where they're going. If you do get lost, well, you're all in it together. From a motivational point of view, you'll find that riding in the company of others spurs you on. Many of your fellow travellers will be on exactly your wavelength. They'll understand why you've taken up cycling and what you're trying to achieve. Their empathy and support can make all the difference.

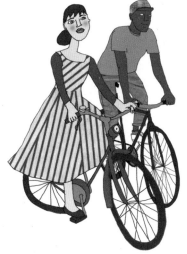

Take time to congratulate yourself when you reach a goal or when you've made significant progress. Savour the moment. If friends praise your achievement and pat you on the back, you're entitled to a glow of pride and to bask in their admiration. In fact, let me be the first to congratulate you and to encourage you to have a small celebration, right now. Why? Because it's all about small steps, remember and, (step one) you've reached the end of this book, (step two) you're thinking about cycling, and (three) you're on your way to improving your health and your life. Keep going – and enjoy the journey!

Acknowledgements.

My thanks to all the individuals and organisations that have provided help and advice in the production of this book, especially:

CTC
Cycling Projects
Dr Adrian Davis
Dr Patrick Guy
Life Cycle UK
London Borough of Croydon
Reading Borough Council
Sustrans
City of York Council

Further information

The UK has three national cycling organisations, British Cycling, CTC and Sustrans. They have helpful full-time staff whose job is to deal with inquires from members of the public. If you have a cycle-related question they're good places to start. Between them, they know just about everything!

These organisations exist to get cycling a better deal. They raise awareness, improve infrastructure, run practical projects and lobby for more favourable legislation. With more members they can be even more effective. You might consider joining one of them (or all three) and adding your support.

British Cycling Stuart Street Manchester M11 4DQ Tel: 0161 274 2046 Email: lovecycling@britishcycling.org.uk Web: www.britishcycling.org.uk	British Cycling is the national governing body for cycle racing in Great Britain and much of their efforts go into promoting the sporty side of cycling. But they're also keen to help more people use bikes for everyday trips. They run a cycle training programme for young people called Go-Ride and they're the organising force behind the popular Sky Rides and Breeze programme (see below).
CTC Parklands Railton Road Guildford Surrey GU2 9JX Tel: 0844 736 8450 or 01483 238 337 (local rate) Email: cycling@ctc.org.uk Web: www.ctc.org.uk	Originally called the Cyclists' Touring Club, these days they're just known by their initials: CTC. They lobby government for policy changes that will encourage more cycling, run promotional projects and provide services to members such as insurance and travel information. There's also a nationwide network of local groups that run regular recreational bike rides.

Sustrans
2 Cathedral Square
College Green
Bristol
BS1 5DD
Tel: 0117 926 8893
Email: reception@sustrans.org.uk
Web: www.sustrans.org.uk

Short for sustainable transport, Sustrans are a charity dedicated to the promotion of walking, cycling and the use of public transport. Their flagship project is the National Cycle Network, which has given us more than 14,000 miles of cycle routes throughout the UK.

Cycling organisations (local)

Cycle Nation
54-57 Allison Street
Digbeth
Birmingham
B5 5TH
Web: www.cyclenation.org.uk

Most major towns and cities have a local cycling campaign. Cyclenation is their umbrella organisation that enables all the groups to speak with a united voice and represents them at the national and international level. Get in touch to find your local campaign group.

London Cycling Campaign
2 Newhams Row
London
SE1 3UZ
Tel: 020 7234 9310
Email: info@lcc.org.uk
Web: www.lcc.org.uk

With 12,000 members, London Cycling Campaign is the largest such organisation in the UK and arguably the most professional. Their mission is to transform the capital into a city where cycling is a safe, easy and convenient travel option for just about everyone.

Cycling clubs and ride opportunities

Bike Week
Web: www.bikeweek.org.uk

Bike Week, usually in June, is an annual celebration of pedal power with events designed to give people a taste of cycling. All over the country there are rides, talks, treasure hunts, bike workshops, carnivals, and cycling fashion shows. Many employers enter in the spirit by offering staff who bike to work a free breakfast.

Breeze Web: www.goskyride.com/ContactUs	Breeze is a programme of activities designed to get more women cycling. A network of Breeze champions organises enjoyable, relaxing, confidence-boosting rides. Rides go at a speed that suits everyone, and they often start or finish at a café so everyone can refresh and chat. The Breeze website has a "find a ride near you" function and lists "female-friendly bike shops."
British Cycling (see above)	The website includes a "club finder" function.
The Canal & River Trust Tel: 0303 040 4040 E-mail: customer.services@ canalrivertrust.org.uk Web: www.canalrivertrust.org.uk	Custodian of many of the nation's canals and rivers. See Chapter Seven.
Clarion Club Web: www.clarioncc.org	With more than 1,000 members in 28 areas the Clarion Club is one the country's biggest cycling clubs. It was born more than 100 years ago as a radical socialist cycling club. Today, the emphasis is less on politics and more on friendship, fun and great bike rides.
CTC (see above)	CTC has hundreds of local groups across the UK offering thousands of rides and events for all abilities. You don't have to be a member to join a ride.

Forestry Commission (England)   See Chapter Seven.
620 Bristol Business Park
Coldharbour Lane
Bristol
BS16 1EJ
Tel: 0300 067 4321
Email: fe.england@forestry.gsi.gov.uk
Web: www.forestry.gov.uk

Forestry Commission (Scotland)   See Chapter Seven.
Silvan House
231 Corstorphine Road
Edinburgh
EH12 7AT
Tel: 0300 067 6156
Email: fcscotland@forestry.gsi.gov.uk
Web: www.scotland.forestry.gov.uk

National Trust   See Chapter Seven.
PO Box 574
Manvers
Rotherham
S63 3FH
Tel: 0844 800 1895 or 0344 800 1895
Email: enquiries@nationaltrust.org.uk
Web: www.nationaltrust.org.uk

The National Trust for Scotland   See Chapter Seven.
Hermiston Quay
5 Cultins Rd
Edinburgh
EH11 4DF
Tel: 0844 493 2100
Email: information@nts.org.uk
Web: www.nts.org.uk

Natural Resources Wales
Ty Cambria
29 Newport Road
Cardiff
CF24 0TP
Tel: 0300 065 3000
Email: enquiries@naturalresourceswales.gov.uk
Web: www.naturalresourceswales.gov.uk/forestry

The forestry authority for Wales. See Chapter Seven.

Northern Ireland Forest Service
Dundonald House
Upper Newtownards Road
Belfast
BT4 3SB
Tel: 0300 200 7852
Email: dardhelpline@dardni.gov.uk
Web: www.dardni.gov.uk/forestry

See Chapter Seven.

Ordnance Survey
Web: www.ordnancesurvey.co.uk

Maps galore, in both paper and electronic format. See Chapter Seven.

Sky Rides
Web: www.goskyride.com

Sky Rides are the brainchild of British Cycling (see above) and Sky (the satellite TV people). The aim is to get a million people – all ages, all abilities – onto their bikes and cycling regularly. There are short neighbourhood rides designed to show people their local area and introduce them to like-minded people, and large scale events in town and city centres that have been closed to motor traffic. It's free of charge to take part, but you need to register in advance.

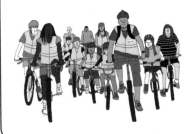

| Tandem Club
Web: www.tandem-club.org.uk | Get in touch to learn more about tandems, or to join a tandem ride. If you have a friend or family member who's unable to ride a regular bike, being a back-rider on a tandem may be a possibility. The website has a useful "tandeming with a disability" section and the club produces a bi-monthly talking journal on CD for visually impaired people. |

Cycle skills training

| Bikeability
Web: https://bikeability.dft.gov.uk/
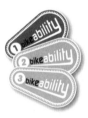 | Bikeability is the "cycling proficiency for the 21st Century." It's all about giving cyclists the knowledge, skills and confidence to cycle safely on today's roads. Most children can get Bikeability training at school either free of charge or at a low cost. Bikeability is for adults too. The website has a "Bikeability near you" function that enables you to find a local provider. |

Inclusive cycling

| CTC (see above) | The website's "inclusive cycling" section covers matters such as tricycles, tandems, hand-powered cycles, and wheelchair cycles, as well as a directory of centres that specialise in helping people with mental or physical disabilities try cycling. |

Cycling Projects
3 Priory Court
Buttermarket Street
Warrington
WA1 2NP
Tel: 01925 234 213
Email ian.tierney@cycling.org.uk
Web: www.cycling.org.uk

Cycling Projects are experts in helping people with health issues take up cycling. They set up the amazing "Wheels for All" network of centres that runs cycling activities for people with disabilities or special needs.

Life Cycle UK
The CREATE Centre
Bristol
BS1 6XN
Tel: 0117 353 4580
Email: office@lifecycleuk.org.uk
Web: www.lifecycleuk.org.uk

Life Cycle runs projects that make cycling accessible to as many people as possible, including "Silver Cyclists" (for older people) "Bike Minded" (for people with mental health issues) and "Two's Company" (tandem rides for people who are blind or sight-impaired).

Other useful sources of help and information

A to B
40 Manor Road
Dorchester
DT1 2AX
Tel: 01305 259998
Email: atob@atob.org.uk
Web: www.atob.org.uk

Magazine specialising in folding bikes and electric bikes. The website has detailed buyers' guides and price comparisons.

ETA
(Environmental Transport Association)
68 High Street
Weybridge
KT13 8RS
0333 000 1234
Web: www.eta.co.uk

A Green version of the AA or RAC. Provides cycle insurance and runs a roadside recovery service for cyclists.

Velo Vision

York Eco Business Centre

Amy Johnson Way

Clifton Moor

York

YO30 4AG

Tel: 01904 692800

Email: howard@velovision.com

Web: www.velovision.com

Magazine specialising in folding bikes, electric bikes and cycles for people with disabilities. The website has two comprehensive "special needs buyer's guides" available as downloads.